Consent
in
Clinical Practice

Margaret Mayberry

with

John Mayberry

RADCLIFFE MEDICAL PRESS

Radcliffe Medical Press Ltd
18 Marcham Road
Abingdon
Oxon OX14 1AA
United Kingdom

www.radcliffe-oxford.com
The Radcliffe Medical Press electronic catalogue and online ordering facility.
Direct sales to anywhere in the world.

British Library Cataloguing in Publication Data

A catalogue record for this book is available from the British Library.

ISBN 1 85775 804 8

Typeset by Joshua Associates Ltd, Oxford
Printed and bound by TJ International Ltd, Padstow, Cornwall

Contents

Preface

Every day doctors and nurses treat patients. Increasing concern about clinical competence requires more detailed patient information about complications and risks of treatment. Control has passed from the professional to the empowered patient, and for many doctors and nurses this is hard to accept. However, developments in English law support these changes.

My interest in consent was fostered by the staff of Cardiff Law School. This ultimately led to the submission of a thesis on the subject, the contents of which form the basis of the larger part of this book. I would especially like to thank Ms Jackie Davies for her support during the writing of my thesis. With encouragement from my husband I have revised the text in order to make the contents accessible to a wider readership. It will hopefully encourage the development of a more structured approach to consent procedures within hospitals and clinics, and also provide a firmer understanding of the legal background to the growing movement towards informed consent.

Central to the need for clearer and simpler information is the ability to produce easy-to-understand booklets, audio tapes and videos about procedures. I would like to thank my husband, John Mayberry, for his contribution to the chapter on this aspect of consent.

I would also like to thank the editors and publishers of the following articles for permission to reproduce some of the contents of these papers.

- Mayberry MK and Mayberry JF (2001) Towards better informed consent in endoscopy: a study of information and consent processes in gastroscopy and flexible sigmoidoscopy. *Eur J Gastroenterol Hepatol.* **13**: 1467–76.
- Mayberry JF and Mayberry M (1996) Effective instructions for patients. *J R Coll Physicians Lond.* **30**: 205–8.

Margaret Mayberry
March 2003

About the authors

Margaret Mayberry qualified as a State Registered Nurse from the Gwent School of Nursing in 1973. She worked as a ward sister with a special interest in diabetes for some years before becoming actively involved in gastrointestinal research. She was the first nurse to hold a research award from the British Digestive Foundation and in the early 1990s she investigated the training needs of nurses in gastroenterology practice. Margaret had an interest in legal and management issues in nursing practice throughout this time. As a result, she read for an LLM at Cardiff University and was awarded the degree with distinction in 2002.

John Mayberry trained at the Welsh National School of Medicine and qualified in 1976. He subsequently worked in various hospitals in South Wales and Nottingham, before being appointed as a consultant gastro-enterologist in Leicester. His research interests in inflammatory bowel disease and oesophageal disorders led to the award of a DSc in the early 1990s. In more recent years his interests have focused on ethnic minority health and legal aspects of day-to-day medical practice. Like Margaret, he has an LLM from the University of Wales.

The patient is so scared he doesn't know what he is signing.

R Quincy
Chief Deputy LA Medical Examiner
Quincy ME
Episode 124, *A Ghost of a Chance*

Introduction

Consent is now a central issue in clinical practice. Doctors and nurses can no longer impose their views on patients as to what constitutes best care. Rather, they need to have the agreement of patients to any intervention – from a simple physical examination to the most complex surgical procedure. Without this agreement, clinical practitioners are open to allegations of assault. As part of the decision-making process, patients require more and more information about procedures. How risky is it? Does the doctor or nurse have experience in performing the procedure? Are they competent at this particular intervention or do they usually have complications? These are the questions which doctors, nurses and other practitioners will have to face with increasing frequency, and they cannot be ignored. Consent by patients therefore requires three elements, namely 'voluntariness, capacity and knowledge',[1] and 'for a consent to be legally valid, all three must be present'.[1]

The methods by which English courts test for the presence of these elements are different for each element. These variations in assessment of the reality of consent have led to an extensive body of English case law, through which a range of tests have been developed to ensure that patients who agree to procedures have both the capacity and the knowledge to do so. This concept of informed consent was originally developed in the USA, and has not yet been openly accepted within the English judicial system. However, it has had an impact on clinical care, so it is likely to affect future judicial decisions.

Writers on informed consent are either idealists or realists. Idealists tend to be judges or medical ethicists. They are concerned with 'materiality of risk, disclosure, alternatives and causation'.[2] They tend to 'emphasise the qualitative dimension of physician–patient interactions concerning treatment decisions'.[2]

In contrast, realists are usually practising physicians. They often question whether patients really want this kind of dialogue. They doubt whether the gains in patient autonomy 'are worth the additional time, money and needless patient anxiety and confusion that informed consent may entail'.[3]

The tension between these two views of consent forms the basis of this book. It will be investigated through a series of chapters which will deal with the following aspects:

- the ethical concepts underlying consent
- who is competent to give consent
- the need for information
- the views of Government and professional organisations.

A comparison between jurisdictions in the USA and England and Wales will explore their different approach to materiality of risk. The former depends on a patient-oriented standard and the latter on a professional one. The likely impact of new professional standards on this approach to consent in England and Wales will also be considered.

In the final section of the book, the practical problems with regard to consent issues will be investigated and related back to elements of patient autonomy and professional beneficence. The difficulties of identifying the type and level of risk which the average patient and specialist solicitors believe should routinely be disclosed will also be reviewed.

In conclusion, some practical recommendations will be developed for clinicians and assessed in the context of case law in England and Wales. The purpose of this book is to stimulate an awareness among doctors, nurses and other professional groups of the need to be sensitive to the rapid developments in the field of patient consent. This awareness should lead to changes in clinical practice. Hopefully this book will be a clarion call to all practitioners to hasten the day when passive consent gives way to informed decisions by patients. When patients are empowered they will also be responsible – responsible for seeking out information about their disease and its investigation and treatment – and so able to make their own informed choices about their care.

References

1   Brooke H and Barton A (2000) Consent to treatment. In: M Powers and N Harris (eds) *Clinical Negligence*. Butterworths, London.
2   Schuck PH (1994) Rethinking informed consent. *Yale Law J.* **103**: 903.
3   Schuck PH (1994) Rethinking informed consent. *Yale Law J.* **103**: 904.

Chapter 1

The ethical concepts behind consent

Introduction

The emergence of consent procedures as part of medical care has a long history with philosophical, religious and social roots as well as legal components. The literary definition of *consent* includes the following ideas: 'to agree; to give permission; to accede; to comply'.[1]

These are all suggestive of a submissive process – one in which the person allows something to be done to him- or herself. In order for consent to operate within acceptable boundaries, there are broad moral principles which must be considered. Most ethicists consider that these are respect for autonomy, beneficence and justice.[2] Within these concepts, human rights play an important role. Such rights are based on a respect for individuals, and this respect will take the form of 'concern for their welfare and respect for their wishes'.[3] The consent process deals with knowing about treatment, accepting it and also the right to refuse it. These rights and obligations have become important legal issues which have been explored through the courts of North America and Western Europe. In some jurisdictions their emergence has imposed an obligation upon carers to provide information. However, in England and Wales this obligation arises from a duty of care rather than from any right on the part of patients to know about their treatment. The standards by which information disclosure will be judged have been defined by the courts in England and Wales as needing to be comparable to those of other practitioners in the same field of therapeutics.[4,5]

Respect for autonomy

Autonomy requires liberty and the capacity to act. It has been defined as 'personal freedom to make moral choices'.[6]

The right to make decisions concerning oneself is clearly part of the democratic process, and is cherished by most people who live in such societies. In the seventeenth and eighteenth centuries philosophical liberalism recognised the capacity for free decision as a hallmark of humans, and the right to exercise that capacity as a key human right.[7] Clearly such choices can be limited by Government-inspired constraints, particularly if they would have adverse effects on others. This is as true in the area of healthcare as in any other area. For example, in sections 37 and 38 of the Public Health (Control of Diseases) Act 1984, provision is made for the enforced removal and detention of people with respiratory tuberculosis who refuse treatment. These sections do not allow people to be forced to participate in a treatment programme, but they do remove them from society so as to prevent the infection of others. In contrast, respect for the right of autonomous patients to refuse treatment which could prolong their lives, but which has no direct impact on the lives of others, is accepted as morally, ethically and legally acceptable. Such rights to refuse treatment are best recognised among Jehovah's Witnesses, who may refuse blood transfusions, even at the risk of their own death. However, such rights have been carefully monitored in recent years. If there is a suspicion that someone may have been unduly influenced in reaching their decision, then doctors can apply to the courts to overrule it.[8] However, the courts view minors from a different standpoint. For example, M was a gravely ill 15-year-old who was 'overwhelmed by her circumstances',[9] and the courts decided that her refusal to undergo a heart transplant could be overridden. In contrast, minors can make decisions about contraception independent of the views of their parents.[10]

As these cases show, society will place restrictions on the choices that are made by individuals. This is particularly so when the decision could harm others or use up scarce resources (e.g. interferon therapy in cases of multiple sclerosis).[11] However, the right to make choices also puts an onus on those who hold information about investigations and treatments to ensure that adequate information is transmitted to the individual to enable them to have the capacity to make the choice. This disclosure must contain within it the type of information which will allow the patient sufficient understanding to enable them to make a truly informed choice. Once these objectives have been achieved, the patient is no longer powerless and they have the capacity to both give and withhold consent. The obligations of the individual information holder may need to be defined by society so that they are uniform and consistent. With regard to patient autonomy, this type of approach may restore the sense of freedom and self-determination that is so often undermined by illness.

It is at this level that it is important to distinguish between two forms of consent. In the harm avoidance model of informed consent,[12] physicians agree that they must obtain consent because procedures have become much more complex, invasive and thus more dangerous for patients than they were 30 years ago. Most physicians have traditionally adopted the harm avoidance model of consent as standard practice. Here there is a disclosure of risks of treatment, but little attention is given to ensuring that the patient understands their consequences. This form of consent:

> is usually considered to be a mere legal formality of signing a consent form. This formality does not honour and respect a patient's individual and personal autonomy, which is the ultimate purpose of obtaining an informed consent.[12]

Harm avoidance assumes that the patient has the capacity to make a decision between alternatives, but does not always call upon them to do so, as some information is withheld. The basis for withholding the information can be found in the developmental history of consent, and is now encapsulated in the following view:

> A doctor will have to exercise his or her professional skill and judgement in deciding what risks the patient should be warned of and the terms in which the warning should be given.[13]

In the case of *Sidaway*, Browne-Wilkinson J recognised that:

> If the disclosure of the risks results in prejudicing the ability of the doctor to cure and the confidence of the patient in the doctor, the existence of a duty to disclose such risks would positively militate against the main purpose of the relation-ship, a factor not present in relation to disclosure of risks by any other professional adviser.[14]

In contrast, the autonomy-enhancing model of informed consent[12] discloses in detail all of the treatments available to the patient, including their risks and benefits. Its ultimate purpose is as follows:

> to ensure that the patient makes an autonomous, rational, reflective, well-understood decision about a medical procedure

or treatment alternative that s(he) believes will be most beneficial.[12]

Current practice in the USA is to follow an autonomy-enhancing model. In England and Wales, harm avoidance consent has been the model followed until recent times. Support for this approach came from *Sidaway v Board of Governors of the Bethlehem Royal Hospital and Maudsley Hospital and Others.*[15] In this judgement it was held that a simple and general explanation of the nature of an operation was sufficient for the patient to give legally valid consent. Whether this was ethically valid depends on one's view of patient autonomy. More detailed information could cause distress to a patient at a time when he or she would be least able to evaluate it because of pain and anxiety. It was also recognised that a patient cannot complain of any lack of information if they have not asked for it.[15]

In 1985 this case confirmed that:

> *There was no doctrine in English law that the patient was entitled to decide everything, just as there was no concept that the doctor was entitled to decide everything. When telling a patient about an operation, the doctor has to decide what ought to be said and how it should be said. The doctor impliedly contracts to provide such information as to be adequate to enable the patient to reach a balanced and rational judgement.*[15]

The problem lies with how someone can reach a balanced and rational decision when they are in possession of an incomplete set of information. The selection and subsequent withholding of information fits in with the philosophy of 'Doctor knows best'. Such an approach is paternalistic, and is characterised by dealing with patients 'in an authoritarian but benevolent way (e.g. by supplying all their needs but regulating their conduct)'.[6] It focuses on the patient as a sick body in need of help, rather than as a rational person who is able to decide about his or her own care. In this way it reduces respect for that person.

Apart from respect for the person, the other element of autonomy is self-determination. This means that people can act in what they believe are their own best interests. They will know how they will be able to cope with pain and the effect that illness may have on their lifestyle. This knowledge will enable and empower them to make an informed decision about treatment and investigations, provided that they receive comprehensive information from their carers.

Autonomy comes with obligations for the patient. A patient's right to make decisions can in some circumstances be abrogated. This is particularly true when the patient lacks the capacity to make a decision, and when health professionals may be expected to treat the patient in accordance with their best interests. It is also true when public policy requires treatment even if the patient does not want it, as in the case of tuberculosis (Public Health (Control of Diseases) Act 1984). Within these constraints the sanctity of individual choice has been a dominant feature of Western thinking throughout the twentieth century.[16,17] For those who are committed to such a sociological view of society, the need for *informed* consent is simply an extension of these concepts. Katz and Capron[18] have identified the following benefits of this type of approach:

- promotion of individual autonomy
- protection of the patient
- avoidance of fraud and duress
- encouragement of self-scrutiny by medical professionals
- promotion of rational decisions
- involvement of the public.

When these decisions are abandoned to the expert, the patient becomes the subject of medical despotism.[19,20] It is for these reasons that understanding is also important when decisions about interventions are needed.

> *Patients . . . also need to share an understanding with professionals about the terms of authorisation before proceeding. Unless agreement exists about the essential features of what is authorised, there can be no assurance that a patient . . . has made an autonomous decision.*[21]

Within the field of consent, explanation of risk is central to any decision making by patients.

> *Enabling consumers to make their own decisions about the risks they are prepared to take requires that they have sufficient information and understanding to do so. There will, however, be some situations when we don't know what the risk is – too many uncertainties may remain to enable proper quantification and therefore to enable consumers to make an informed choice.*[22]

The role of trust in risk communication has been the subject of recent research, and it is now clear that the message is judged not by the content but by the source. If the source is not trusted, good delivery of the message can be counter-productive.[23]

Trust depends upon 'perceived competence, objectivity, fairness, consistency and goodwill'.[23] The mode of presenting risk can influence patients' understanding and so affect any decisions, thus preventing truly autonomous authorisation.[21]

Beneficence

The recent concerns about clinical care seen in England and Wales, especially with regard to the activities of the general practitioner Harold Shipman, have sharpened anxieties about the clinical practice of doctors and whether these are always beneficial. However, since the time of Hippocrates the moral basis for the practice of medicine has been to help, or at least to do no harm. The principles of non-maleficence and beneficence have four basic elements:[21]

- to inflict no harm
- to prevent harm
- to remove harm
- to promote good.

These elements are not mutually exclusive, although they can sometimes be in conflict. They also include the concept of negligence, where negligence has been defined as 'the absence of due care. In the professions it involves a departure from the professional standards that determine due care in a given set of circumstances'.[21]

This can be either intentional or unintentional, and is usually blameworthy. For physicians, the positive benefit that they should seek is the alleviation of disease and injury and the prolongation or sustaining of life. The harm to be prevented is the pain, suffering and disability of disease.

However, the use of life-sustaining treatments occasionally violates patients' interests, e.g. pain can be so severe and physical restraints so burdensome that these factors outweigh anticipated benefits, such as brief prolongation of life.[21]

In this case, achievement of the objectives of treatment may be through means which could be considered cruel or inhumane. However, the term 'beneficence' includes acts of mercy, kindness and charity, and it concerns the motivation to act in the best interests of others. The goal of medicine is to promote the welfare of patients. Therefore, for clinicians, the risk of harm caused by interventions must be counterbalanced by the possible benefits to patients. In practical terms, the views of patients also enter into this equation, as they may reject a doctor's recommendation.

However, to overrule this refusal of treatment would interfere with the patient's autonomy, and such an approach would be paternalistic.

It is this form of medical paternalism that probably characterised the Hippocratic school:

> concealing most things from the patient . . . sometimes reprove sharply and emphatically, and sometimes comfort with solicitude and attention, revealing nothing of the patient's future or present condition.[24]

The need to avoid harm and do good within the Hippocratic tradition formed the basis for the implicit trust whereby patients were encouraged to 'confidently entrust themselves to him for treatment'.[24] The tension between beneficence and patient autonomy has been recognised by Beauchamp and Childress:

> Whether respect for the autonomy of patients should have priority over professional beneficence directed at those patients is a central problem in biomedical ethics.[21]

It was not until the middle of the sixth century AD in Italy that patients were encouraged to question their physicians: 'let the patient ask you about his ailment and hear from you the truth about it'.[25]

However, such attitudes were uncommon, and throughout most of antiquity and the Middle Ages the physician was expected to provide the patient with the best treatment available, and this was to be accepted by the patient without question. Beauchamp and Childress have summarised the situation as follows:

> Beneficence provides the primary goal and rationale of medicine and health care, whereas respect for autonomy . . . and justice sets moral limits on the professional's actions in pursuit of this goal.[21]

A specific effect of beneficence on the provision of information has been the traditional attitude adopted by many clinicians when they have argued that disclosure of certain types of information can cause harm to patients. An ethical approach to care requires them to avoid doing this.[21,26] A problem also arises with regard to the conflict between beneficence and a patient's refusal of treatment which is in their best interest. This may be due to incomplete information, or it may reflect an autonomous decision. In practice, autonomy and beneficence can coincide or may be at distinct ends of a range of options.

Justice

Social co-operation between individuals means that people will be treated with fairness. Justice is concerned with fairness, equitability and appropriate treatment of people. It means that individuals will receive goods, service or information to which they are entitled.[21] Distributive justice concerns the distribution of all rights and responsibilities in society. If it is difficult to exercise this right or responsibility, this represents an injustice, and an example is the failure to share with the patient accurate facts concerning their condition and proposed investigations and remedies. Failure to share facts means that the patient cannot make rational decisions. However, an ethical difficulty concerns how much information should be given to ensure adequate understanding by the patient about the issues of need for diagnosis and treatment as well as the risks of procedures and treatment. The decision as to how much information should be given to patients is ultimately made by society, and in this case 'justice is located in the guarantee that services will be provided to fulfil a particular community-endorsed conception of social goals'.[21]

From this information, patients will need to know the likely outcomes of their choices. The benefits of such an approach have been clarified by Katz and Capron.[18]

Justice requires the fair distribution of healthcare to everyone. During the past decade some attention has been focused on the effects of race and gender on delivery of healthcare. Studies among Asian patients with cardiac disease in the UK have shown that they have less access to investigations such as stress tests[27] and to more invasive procedures such as coronary angiography.[28] Justice requires that patients from minority groups receive adequate information about procedures and treatments. Clearly this needs to be presented in a form which can be understood.

In summary, there is a tension between the beneficence of healthcare professionals, the autonomous decisions of patients and the community's need to keep society healthy. The balance between these and the scarcity of medical resources is a dilemma which distributive justice should be able to address. However, to do this:

> It may well be both justifiable and wise to remedy, where possible, both the defects of reasoning and of information which militate against the individual's capacity for autonomy. The reasons for doing so would not be that such

action was in the individual's own interests, but rather that it was in the interests of us all.[3]

Although the primary decision about medical investigation and treatment belongs with patients, the courts provide a balance by helping to identify the standards of disclosure which doctors and other paramedical practitioners should follow. Much of the current debate around consent is concerned with the degree and nature of disclosure. Fletcher has defined consent as affecting 'our relations with others by vesting in them the power to act toward us in ways that would otherwise be wrong and prohibited'.[29]
  For Fletcher:

> *Consent is not valid for either of its functions (undermining the harm, negating the right to complain) unless it is freely and intelligently given. The consenting party must know the relevant facts and act without being under pressure.*[29]

Such an interpretation lends strength to the argument that patients are entitled to a full disclosure about the nature of investigations and treatment, including the failure to conduct them. Although the concept of 'informed consent' in the American meaning of those words is foreign to English law, Lord Reid recognised that:

> *English law goes to great lengths to protect a person of full age and capacity from interference with his personal liberty . . . . So it would be unwise to make even minor concessions.*[30]

Recent guidelines from the Department of Health are unequivocal:

> *If an adult with capacity makes a voluntary and appropriately informed decision to refuse treatment, this decision must be respected . . . This is the case even where this may result in the death of the person/and or the death of an unborn child, whatever the stage of the pregnancy.*[31]

Central to this thinking and the General Medical Council guidelines[32] is the provision of adequate information to allow patients to make autonomous decisions. The underlying philosophy that pervades some guidelines on consent is that if sufficient easy-to-understand information is given to patients, they will choose the best treatment. Justice requires that this information is unbiased and includes details of the adverse consequences of various treatments.

References

1 Schwarz C (ed.) (1994) *The Chambers Dictionary*. Chambers Harrap Publishers Ltd, Edinburgh.

2 Faden R, Beauchamp TL and King NMP (1986) *A History and Theory of Informed Consent*. Oxford University Press, New York.

3 Harris J (1985) *The Value of Life. An introduction to medical ethics*. Routledge, London.

4 *Bolam v Friern Hospital Management Committee* [1957] 1 WLR 582.

5 *Bolitho v City and Hackney Health Authority* [1993] 4 Med LR 381 (CA).

6 (1984) *Longman Dictionary of the English Language*. Longman, Harlow.

7 Polani P (1983) The development of the concepts and practice of patient consent. In: GR Dunstan and MJ Seller (eds) *Consent in Medicine. Convergence and divergence in tradition*. King Edward's Hospital Fund for London, London.

8 *Re T (adult medical treatment without consent)* [1992] 4 All ER 649 CA 30/7/92.

9 *Re M (a minor) (medical treatment) sub nom. In the matter of the inherent jurisdiction sub nom re M (child: refusal of medical treatment)* [1999] LTL 15/7/1999 2 FLR 1097 [1999]: [2000] 52 BMLR 124 p. 1 and 2 of Document No. C7200105 (Lawtel).

10 *Gillick v West Norfolk and Wisbech Area Health Authority* [1986] AC 112.

11 Hawkes N (2001) Nurse of the Year pioneers clinic. *The Times*. **31 October**: 3.

12 Switankowsky IS (1998) *A New Paradigm for Informed Consent*. University Press of America Inc., Lanham, MD, p. 2.

13 HC(90)22 (1990) *A Guide to Consent for Examination or Treatment*. Department of Health, London.

14 *Sidaway v Board of Governors of the Bethlehem Royal Hospital and Maudsley Hospital and Others* [1984] 1 All ER 1018: [1984] QB 493.

15 *Sidaway v Board of Governors of the Bethlehem Royal Hospital and Maudsley Hospital and Others* [1985] AC 871, HL at 871.

16 Durkheim E (1953) *The Division of Labour in Society*. Free Press, Glencoe, IL.

17 Weber M (1956) *The Protestant Ethic and the Spirit of Capitalism*. Scribner's, New York.

18 Katz J and Capron AM (1975) *Catastrophic Diseases: who decides what?* Russell Sage Foundation, New York.

19 Friedson E (1970) *The Profession of Medicine*. Dodd and Mead, New York.

20 Appelbaum PS, Lidz CW and Meisel A (1987) *Informed Consent. Legal theory and clinical practice*. Oxford University Press, New York.

21 Beauchamp TL and Childress JF (2001) *Principles of Biomedical Ethics* (5e). Oxford University Press, Oxford.

22 McKechnie S and Davies S (1999) Consumers and risk. In: P Bennett and K Calman (eds) *Risk Communication and Public Health*. Oxford University Press, Oxford.

23 Bennett P (1999) Understanding responses to risk: some basic findings. In: P Bennett and K Calman (eds) *Risk Communication and Public Health*. Oxford University Press, Oxford.

24 Jones WHS (trans.) (1967) *Hippocrates. Vol. 11. Decorum XVI*. Heinemann, London (quoted in Polani PE (1983) The development of the concepts and practice of patient consent. In: *Convergence and Divergence in Tradition*. King Edward's Hospital Fund for London, London).

25 MacKinney LC (1952) Medical ethics and etiquette in the early middle ages: the persistence of Hippocratic ideals. *Bull History Med.* **26**: 1–31.

26 Henderson LJ (1935) Physician and patient as a social system. *NEJM.* **212**: 819–23.

27 Lear JT, Lawrence IG, Burden AC and Pohl JE (1994) A comparison of stress test referral rates and outcomes between Asians and Europeans. *J R Soc Med.* **87**: 661–2.

28 Trevelyan J, Needham EW, Halim M *et al.* (2001) Evaluation of patient characteristics and utilisation of invasive cardiac procedures in a UK ethnic population with unstable angina pectoris. *Int J Cardiol.* **77**: 275–80.

29 Fletcher GP (1996) *Basic Concepts of Legal Thought*. Oxford University Press, New York.

30 *S v S* [1970] 3 All ER 107 at 111.

31 Department of Health (2001) *Reference Guide to Consent for Examination or Treatment*. Department of Health, London.

32 General Medical Council (undated) *Seeking Patients' Consent: the ethical considerations*. General Medical Council, London.

Chapter 2

Consent to investigation and treatment: who is competent to give consent?

Introduction

The validity of a patient's consent depends on a number of factors. One of these factors, which is central to the process, is the question of a patient's competence. The range of ability among patients follows a continuum from incompetence through to competence. A practical question for clinicians is where on that continuum they must place a marker below which a patient would be unable to give consent because they lacked competence. A simple approach is to suggest that the status of a patient can be used to define whether they have competence. In this situation, minors and those with mental disorders could be said to lack competence. Such approaches have been challenged, and will be reviewed in this chapter. In England and Wales, assessment has been based on capacity, and in practice:

> The right to decide one's own fate presupposes a capacity to do so. Every adult is presumed to have that capacity, but it is a presumption which can be rebutted. This is not a question of the degree of intelligence or education of the adult concerned.[1]

Case law has developed around the status question and has clarified who has competence and how it may be assessed. Most cases have arisen because patients have refused treatment and their clinician or family has challenged their decision.

Refusal of treatment by adults

In *Re F (mental patient: sterilisation)*, Neill J confirmed that:

> The fact that as a general rule the consent of the patient must
> be obtained before any operation or other treatment on his
> body is carried out means that the patient has the right to
> refuse. Moreover, the right to refuse exists even where there are
> overwhelming medical reasons in favour of the treatment, and
> probably even where if the treatment is not carried out the
> patient's life will be at risk.[2]

However, this case concerned a young woman with significant mental
subnormality, and it did not clarify how capacity to give consent should
be defined outside of any mental health legislation.

Re T (adult: refusal of medical treatment)[3] concerned a woman who
was 34 weeks pregnant when she was injured in a car accident. The
question of a blood transfusion arose, but after a private conversation
with her mother, who was a Jehovah's Witness, T told a staff nurse
that although she was no longer active in the sect, she still retained
some of its beliefs and did not want a transfusion. As a result, she
signed a refusal of consent to blood transfusion form. An emergency
Caesarean section became necessary, and following the procedure the
intensive-care-unit consultant felt inhibited about prescribing a blood
transfusion. The patient's father and boyfriend applied to the court for
assistance, and following an emergency hearing the judge authorised a
transfusion.

The Court of Appeal recognised that every adult had the right and
capacity to decide whether to accept medical treatment, even if this led
to permanent injury or death. However, if a person's capacity to make
that decision is lacking, then doctors may disregard such instructions in
the patient's best interests, provided that they have sought a declaration
from the courts as to the lawfulness of the proposed treatment.

Donaldson MR summarised the situation as follows:

> Prima facie every adult has the right and capacity to
> decide whether or not he will accept medical treatment . . .
> Furthermore, it matters not whether the reasons for the refusal
> were rational or irrational, unknown or even non-existent . . .
> However, the presumption of capacity to decide which stems
> from the fact that the patient is an adult, is rebuttable.[4]

Butler-Sloss LJ quoted with approval the view of Robins JA in the
Canadian case of *Malette v Shulman:*

The right to determine what shall be done with one's own body is a fundamental right in our society. The concepts inherent in this right are the bedrock upon which the principles of self-determination and individual autonomy are based.[5,6]

This case centred on the validity of a refusal of consent and the effects of undue influence from the mother. When assessing the capacity of an adult who had refused treatment, doctors were advised to consider the effect of the following:

- shock, pain or drugs
- outside influences
- whether the circumstances had changed and did not apply to the initial decision.

In this case, the Court of Appeal considered that the refusal was invalid because it did not cover the emergency situation which had arisen. The question which may need to be considered is whether the imposing figure of a doctor suggesting an investigation or form of treatment, but only providing incomplete information about risks and complications, may have undue influence over an anxious patient. However, in general doctors should consider most patients to have the capacity to give consent.

Every adult is presumed to have . . . capacity, but it is a presumption which can be rebutted. This is not a question of the degree of intelligence or education of the adult concerned. However, a small minority of the population lack the necessary mental capacity due to mental illness or retarded development.[1]

Tests of capacity were examined in *Re C (adult refusal of treatment)*.[7] At the age of 68 years, C developed gangrene of his foot. The clinicians who were caring for him recommended a below-knee amputation. However, C was a paranoid schizophrenic who believed that he was an internationally respected doctor. He applied for an injunction to prevent the amputation, which was granted by Thorpe J, despite the possibility of death, the probability of which was rated as high as 85%. The reasoning behind this decision centred around the question of whether, despite his schizophrenia, C was able to 'understand the *nature, purpose* and *effects* of the proferred amputation'[7] (*italic emphasis added*).

Dr Eastman, who was an expert witness in the case, suggested the following three-stage test of capacity:

- comprehension and retention of information
- believing the information
- ability to weigh the information in the balance and make a choice.

The patient needs to be able to show discretion and discrimination in his or her use of information. Although this is a test of capacity to understand, and not of actual understanding, it is difficult to see how someone could weigh information in the balance without understanding or comprehending it. Indeed this is the first stage of Dr Eastman's test, and it is not always given appropriate weight. This decision upheld C's autonomy and considered it to be of greater importance than where his clinical best interests lay.

In relation to this case, Kennedy and Grubb made the following suggestion:

> It must, therefore, be the law that competence is determined by reference to the unvarying conceptual standard of capacity or ability to understand. Whether therefore a patient who is judged competent because she has the capacity or ability to understand, in fact consented, is a distinct question turning upon the reality of the consent based upon legally adequate information.[8]

In relation to mental health issues, the Mental Health Act Code of Practice suggests that:

> a The assessment of capacity . . . should be made with a specific proposal of treatment in mind.
> b This assessment needs to be made at the time that the treatment is proposed.[9]

Although these comments are directed at patients with mental health issues, they do provide some suggestions as to when and in which situations capacity should be tested. This is a later topic of this book, when patients' comprehension, retention and ability to weigh information before giving consent to endoscopic procedures are considered and tested in a formal way. These three elements constitute a patient's capacity to understand legally adequate information, which is what the law requires. It was W's failure to comprehend and retain information and balance it in reaching a decision that led Johnson J to give authority to an obstetrician to end her labour.[10]

In *Re MB (Caesarean section)*,[11] the key factors of capacity and consent were reviewed and the potential impact of the Convention on Human Rights was considered. MB had been advised to undergo a Caesarean section, as this would substantially improve her child's chances of survival. Despite giving consent to the surgery, MB repeatedly withdrew it because of an irrational fear of needles. An application was made for a declaration that it would be lawful to operate and to use reasonable force to achieve this objective if necessary. A psychiatrist stated that:

> the appellant lacked the capacity to see beyond the immediate situation of proximity to a needle, although she clearly understood the need for a Caesarean procedure.[11]

The Court of Appeal confirmed that a pregnant woman is entitled to the same degree of autonomy as anyone else, and that she can refuse treatment for any rational or irrational reason, or indeed for no reason at all. However, it supported Hollis J's decision that the Caesarean section should go ahead. It held that:

> (6) A person lacked capacity if some impairment or disturbance of mental functioning rendered the person unable to make a decision whether to consent to or refuse a treatment.
> (7) Temporary factors may completely erode capacity, but must have done so to the extent that the ability to decide is completely absent. Fear and panic may also destroy the capacity to make a decision.[11]

The Court decided that MB was temporarily incompetent because of her fear of needles, which dominated her thinking and prevented her considering anything else. This led her to refuse surgery. Such cases as *Re MB (Caesarean section)*[11] have broadened the nature of the test in *Re C.*[7] Panic, indecisiveness and irrationality do not as such amount to incompetence, but they may be symptoms or evidence of lack of competence. *Re C (adult refusal of treatment)*[7] and *Re MB (Caesarean section)*[11] appear to differ in that the consequences of refusal in the former case could have been the death of C, whereas in the latter case it would have been the death of MB and her child. Although Butler-Sloss LJ emphasised that the consequences of refusal were not the basis for the court's decision, some might consider that a link is beginning to emerge.

Consent to treatment and refusal by minors

A status approach would hold that minors do not have the capacity either to give consent to treatment or to refuse it. However, with the changing social status of young people, their involvement in treatment decisions became inevitable at the end of the twentieth century. At this time the Department of Health and Social Security issued guidance on contraception and children under the age of 16 years. Their advice was that in exceptional cases 'it was for a doctor to decide whether to prescribe contraception without informing the parents of the child'.[12]

Mrs Gillick sought a declaration that such advice was unlawful. Woolf J refused her application, but the Court of Appeal agreed to it. However, the House of Lords allowed the appeal by the Department of Health and Social Security by a majority of 3 to 2. The issue of consent was central to their discussions, and Lord Fraser's view was that:

> *It seems to me verging on the absurd to suggest that a boy or a girl aged 15 could not effectively consent, for example, to have a medical examination of some trivial injury to his body or even to have a broken arm set . . . Provided the patient, whether a boy or a girl, is capable of understanding what is proposed, and of expressing his or her own wishes, I see no good reason for holding that he or she lacks the capacity to express them validly and effectively and to authorise the medical man to make the examination or give the treatment which he advises.*[13]

Lord Scarman made it clear that the age from which a person can give consent should be:

> *if and when the child achieves sufficient understanding and intelligence to enable him or her to understand fully what is proposed. It will be a question of fact whether a child seeking advice has sufficient understanding of what is involved to give a consent valid in law.*[13]

Although this case makes it clear that a child may have the capacity to give consent, this has not applied to the withholding of consent or refusal of treatment. The decisions by young people to refuse treatment have been regularly overridden,[14,15] and this contrasts with the situation among adults, unless they are considered to be subject to undue influence which has led them to refuse treatment. This approach was particularly well demonstrated in *Re M (a minor) (medical treatment) sub nom in the matter of the inherent jurisdiction sub nom Re M (child: refusal of medical treatment).*[16] M was a 15-year-old girl who refused to undergo cardiac transplantation. She felt that she would 'rather die than have the transplant and have someone else's heart'.[16]

In addition, she did not wish to take immunosuppressive medication for the rest of her life. However, M's mother consented to the surgery on her behalf, and an application was made to the court to override M's decision. The opinion of the Official Solicitor, on behalf of M, was that although she was an intelligent person and her views should carry considerable weight, she was overwhelmed by the circumstances and the nature of the decision and so lacked the capacity to make a decision. Johnson J agreed and on the basis of 'seeking to achieve what was best for M'[16] gave authority for the operation. This case very clearly confirms the reluctance of the courts to support a refusal of treatment by a minor, and this needs to be compared with their support for independent action when consenting to something as first conceptualised in *Gillick v West Norfolk and Wisbech AHA*.[13]

Consent to treatment, capacity and linguistic skills

Central to the concept of capacity to give consent is the ability to comprehend and retain information about treatment. The ability to comprehend information will depend upon the patient's ability to understand the language. When a patient uses a language other than English on a day-to-day basis, they may have difficulties in understanding information about tests and procedures. There have been no medical cases to date which have focused on a patient's lack of capacity to give consent because they did not understand English. However, there have been cases where contracts have been declared void on this basis.[17,18] The signing of clinical consent forms by patients who are not fluent in English, and the use of non-professional translators, such as hospital porters, family or friends could equally be regarded as void. Later in this book the understanding of an information sheet for patients among ethnic groups will be considered. Similar difficulties can arise when someone is illiterate.[19] The relevance of *Lloyds Bank plc v Waterhouse*[19] to patients with poor reading skills or lack of English is obvious. The clinician has a duty to answer any questions clearly and to ensure that they are understood.

Capacity and understanding

Kennedy and Grubb have raised an interesting question about the nature of understanding:

> *If the test of understanding is actual understanding . . . then whether or not the girl understands and therefore is competent*

to consent may turn on what she is told. Indeed, this seems to have been Lord Donaldson's approach in Re R (a minor) (wardship: consent to treatment) [1991] . . . If the girl is not given certain information, she may not understand enough, but this would not be the product of any lack of competence but merely that she decided in ignorance. It would be an unsatisfactory state of law if doctors could be controlling the information given to a patient and thereby grant or deny her competence . . . It must, therefore, be the law that competence is determined by reference to the unvarying conceptual standard of capacity or ability to understand.[8]

The consequence of such thinking is that if a patient fails to understand the information that is given to him or her, further explanation will be mandatory before seeking his or her consent to the procedure. It also has direct consequences for patients who clearly have capacity, but who cannot understand the information because of literacy problems or linguistic difficulties. The empirical study reported at the end of this book considers ways in which understanding can be checked, thereby opening up the possibility of further clarification by a clinician.

References

1 *Re T (adult: refusal of treatment)* [1993] Fam 95 at 112–113.

2 *Re F (mental patient: sterilisation)* [1990] 2 AC 1, HL at 29.

3 *Re T (adult: refusal of medical treatment)* [1992] 4 All ER 649.

4 *Re T (adult: refusal of medical treatment)* [1992] 4 All ER 649 at 650.

5 *Re T (adult: refusal of medical treatment)* [1992] 4 All ER 649 at 665.

6 *Malette v Shulman* [1990] 72 (OR 92d) 417 at 432.

7 *Re C (adult refusal of treatment)* [1994] 1 WLR 290. Quoted in Stauch M and Wheat K with Tingle J (1998) *Sourcebook on Medical Law.* Cavendish Publishing Ltd, London.

8 Kennedy I and Grubb A (1994) *Medical Law* (2e). Butterworths, London.

9 *Mental Health Act (1983) Code of Practice,* paragraph 15.10.

10 *Norfolk and Norwich Healthcare (NHS) Trust v W* [1996] 2 FLR 613.

11 *Re MB (Caesarean section)* [1997] LTL 26/3/97: ILR 8/4/97: TLR 18/4/97: [1997] 2 FLR 426: [1997] FCR 541: [1998] 38 BMLR 175.

12 Stauch M and Wheat K with Tingle J (1998) *Sourcebook on Medical Law.* Cavendish Publishing Ltd, London.

13 *Gillick v West Norfolk and Wisbech AHA* [1986] 1 AC 112, HL (Fraser,

Scarman, Bridge, Brandon and Templeman LL). Quoted in Stauch M and Wheat K with Tingle J (1998) *Sourcebook on Medical Law*. Cavendish Publishing Ltd, London.

14 *Re R (a minor) (wardship: consent to treatment)* [1992] Fam 11, [1991] 4 All ER 177 CA [1992] 7.

15 *Re W (a minor) (medical treatment)* [1992] 4 All ER 627, CA [1992] 9 BMLR 22.

16 *Re M (a minor) (medical treatment) sub nom in the matter of the inherent jurisdiction sub nom Re M (child: refusal of medical treatment)* [1999] LTL 15/7/1999: [2000] 52 BMLR 124: [1999] 2 FLR 1097.

17 *Kunnath v The State* [1993] 4 All ER 30: [1993] 1 WLR 1315: [1993] 98 CAR 455: Guardian 20/8/93 [1993] 137 SJ(LB) 195: [1993] 143 NLJ 1332: TLR 30/7/93 Lawtel Document No. C0000007. Kunnath was convicted in Mauritius, where the proceedings were conducted in English. He stated from the dock that he did not understand what was being said. It was held that: 'the conduct of proceedings could not be said to have had a fair trial'. His conviction was quashed.

18 *Hamid Dedsahti Haghighat v (1) Abdul Razzak Mohammed Rakim Baksh (2) James Hebblethwaite and Baksh (a firm) (3) Djaved Sepjani (4) Chatwani and Co (a firm): Solicitors' Indemnity Fund (substituted for TSB Bank plc) v (1) Djaved Sepjani (2) Hamid Dedsahti Haghighat* [1999] LTL 27/10/99 Extempore (unreported elsewhere) Document No. C8400534. The Court of Appeal upheld the decision of the original judge that the transfer of a lease, which had been obtained by fraud, was void. The respondent was Iranian and illiterate, and the transfer of the lease had been 'procured without his knowledge or consent at a time when he could not read, speak or understand English'.

19 *Lloyds Bank plc v Waterhouse* [1990] ILR 27/2/90: [1991] 10 Tr LR: [1992] 2 FLR 97: [1991] 2 Fam Law 23. An illiterate farmer signed an all-moneys guarantee in respect of a bank loan to his son. Although he asked the bank about the terms, he was too shy to tell them he could not read, but the answers were inadequate. The Court of Appeal held that he had no duty to disclose his illiteracy, and his appeal was allowed.

Chapter 3

Consent to investigation and treatment: the need for information

Introduction

In 1985, in *Mishap or Malpractice*, Clifford Hawkins wrote 'The consent issue *by itself* is unlikely to be a legal problem for the doctor'.[1] However, in subsequent years the importance of consent has increased, and it is now central to many legal and ethical issues in medicine. There has been a policy movement towards patient empowerment, which can only be achieved through adequate and comprehensive information.

This need to obtain permission to investigate and treat patients has emerged over recent centuries in England and Wales. Initially, skilled clinicians needed protection from accusations of unwanted touching, which would have brought them within the compass of either criminal battery or the tort of trespass. Changes in the nature of permission have developed as clinicians have become less distant and patients have become more informed and assertive. In this chapter, the role of case law in these developments in England and Wales will be explored and compared with other jurisdictions.

Acceptance of provision of information and consent to treatment as standard practices

In 1767, Slater took action against Baker, a surgeon from St Bartholomew's Hospital, and Stapleton, an apothecary, for their poor clinical management of his fractured leg.[2] The plaintiff had sent for Stapleton to remove the bandage from his leg. However, rather than doing so he sought help from Baker and rebroke the patient's leg. In the view of the court they had:

> *so ignorantly and unskilfully treated the plaintiff, that they ignorantly and unskilfully broke and disunited the callous of the plaintiff's leg after it was set.*[3]

The views of other surgeons were that this was the wrong procedure to employ at this stage of recovery. Even if such an approach had been correct these surgeons would not have proceeded without the consent of the patient, and its lack was seen as unacceptable:

> *All the surgeons said they never do anything of this kind without consent, and if this plaintiff should not be content with the present damages, but bring another action of trespass.*[4]

Lord Chief Justice Wilmot summed up the rules of consent in a way that is still largely true today:

> *consent; this is the usage and law of surgeons . . . and it is reasonable that a patient should be told what is about to be done to him.*[5]

Slater v Baker and Stapleton (1767)[2] confirmed the traditional approach that clinicians must obtain permission from their patients to undertake procedures, and that it was reasonable the patient should be told about what was to be done. Further developments with regard to the issue of consent took place mainly in the USA, but it was not until the twentieth century that clearer legal definitions emerged. Some of this discussion revolved around the distinction between battery and negligence, while in the USA a fiduciary relationship between doctors and patients was accepted. Although cases from the USA carry no authority in England and Wales, they have often been used to inform legal discussion here, as well as in other jurisdictions.

The initial cases in the USA which dealt with inadequate consent were grounded in battery. The best known example is *Schloendorff v The Society of the New York Hospitals.*[6] In this case a tumour was removed surgically from Mary Schloendorff when she was anaesthetised. This was done without her consent or knowledge. The first court found in her favour, and this judgement was upheld on appeal. Judge Benjamin Cardozo recognised that:

> *The wrong complained of is not merely negligence. It is trespass. Every human being of adult years and sound mind has a right to determine what shall be done with his own*

body, and a surgeon who performs an operation without his patient's consent commits an assault, for which he is liable in damages.[6]

In Katz's view, *Schloendorff v The Society of the New York Hospitals*[6] did not establish 'patients' rights to "thoroughgoing self-determination" in interactions with their physicians'.[7]

The case was concerned with torts committed by surgeons using the New York Hospital's facilities. It did not consider the information needs of the patient, or even whether there had been a violation of informed consent. However, Cardozo's opinion is widely quoted and has been considered in cases from many jurisdictions, including that of England and Wales.[8]

It was in 1957 that the term 'informed consent' first emerged in California in *Salgo v Leland Stanford Junior University Board of Trustees.*[9] Martin Salgo developed permanent paralysis following translumbar aortography. He sued his physicians for negligence in the performance of the procedure, and for failing to warn him of the risks. In this case, Justice Bray in the California Court of Appeals took up the *amicus* brief submitted by the American College of Surgeons in support of the defendants. Ironically, Justice Bray used it to support his view that:

A physician violates his duty to his patient and subjects himself to liability if he withholds any facts which are necessary to form the basis of an intelligent consent by the patients to the proposed treatment.[9]

However, he tempered this decision by saying that full disclosure must be balanced by clinical discretion as to what might alarm an apprehensive patient. This case extended a doctor's duty beyond disclosing the nature and consequences of treatment to include disclosure of risks and alternative forms of treatment, and limited the concept of therapeutic privilege. The court thus created the concept of 'informed consent'. Interestingly, the core of Justice Bray's definition of 'informed consent' came from the American College of Surgeons through the brief which they submitted to the court.[7] The parallel with the current situation in England and Wales, where 'informed consent' is being promoted by the Department of Health, the Royal Colleges and other medical groups, is striking. Just as Justice Bray opened up the issue of how much freedom of choice to grant to patients, these organisations are now doing so in England and Wales. The recommendations from the Bristol Inquiry are also in line with these developments.

The next major legal aspect of consent in England and Wales was the definition of its scope. In jurisdictions such as the USA, this was intimately associated with the development of the 'informed consent' doctrine. Although this doctrine has been consistently rejected in England and Wales, subsequent discussion will confirm that many elements have been accepted in practice.

The scope of consent

In *Breen v Baker* in 1956, Mrs Breen agreed to a dilatation and curettage and signed a consent form which stated 'I agree to leave the nature and extent of the operation to be performed to the discretion of the surgeon'.[10]

However, Mr Baker actually performed a total hysterectomy. Mrs Breen's claim of battery failed because of the nature of the consent that she had given. Such wide consent continues to be embodied in many consent forms, including those issued by the NHS Management Executive from 1990, which contained the following wording:

> *I understand that any procedure in addition to the investigation or treatment described on this form will only be carried out if it is necessary and in my best interests and can be justified for medical reasons.*[11]

Until very recently, Mrs Breen might still have undergone a hysterectomy unless she had:

> *told the doctor . . . about any additional procedures I would not wish to be carried out straightaway without my having the opportunity to consider them first.*[11]

More recently, in *Christine Williamson v East London and the City Health Authority and Others*,[12] £20 000 damages were awarded for medical negligence when a surgeon performed a mastectomy rather than replacing a breast prosthesis. The surgeon had not obtained written consent, although she recalled saying to the plaintiff that her intentions were to do more than was originally planned. It was held that the surgeon did not properly inform the patient of her plan to increase the magnitude of the operation, and that Ms Williamson had not consented to such an extensive operation.

Between 1956 and 1998 the scope of consent had become largely limited to specific procedures discussed with the patient. The existence of 'catch-all' sections[11] in some consent forms is unlikely to provide protection against actions in negligence or battery. With patient empowerment there has been a movement away from opting out of procedures and towards opting into them. This approach is consistent with current standards of care in England and Wales.

In the USA, in *Natanson v Kline* (1960)[13] in 1960 the court grounded 'informed consent liability in negligence rather than battery'.[8]

In this case, Mrs Irma Natanson suffered cobalt therapy burns as a result of treatment aimed at reducing the risk of recurrence of breast cancer. The choice of negligence as a basis for dealing with inadequate consent placed on plaintiffs the additional need to prove that they would have refused the proposed treatment if they had been fully informed. In addition, Justice Schroeder continued to accept the following:

> *The duty of the physician to disclose, however, is limited to those disclosures which a reasonable medical practitioner would make under the same or similar circumstances.*[13]

He based these views on Dr Hubert Smith's article on 'Therapeutic privilege to withhold specific diagnosis from patient sick with serious or fatal disease'.[14] They recognised the same guidelines for information as applied to investigations and treatments. As a result, many subsequent cases have followed a similar route because of the apparent ease of applying what in England and Wales might have been described as the Bolam principle. This need for the plaintiff to prove that they would have refused treatment has been seen in a wide range of jurisdictions (e.g. *Hills v Potter & Anor*[15] in England and Wales, *Rosenberg v Percival*[16] in Australia and *Walsh v Irish Family Planning Services*[17] in Eire).

The level of risk which should be disclosed

In 1956, John Bolam sued Friern Hospital Management Committee[18] because of negligent treatment which he had received in 1954. He had suffered from depression and was admitted as a voluntary patient to Friern Hospital, where he was prescribed electroconvulsive therapy (ECT). The grounds for his claim included 'failing to warn him of the risks involved in the treatment'.[18]

It had been his doctors' practice 'not to warn their patients of the risks of the treatment (which they believed to be small) unless asked; if asked, they said that there was a very slight risk'.[18]

In this case, McNair established the standards by which clinical practice would be judged. It became known as the Bolam principle:

> *The test is the standard of the ordinary skilled man exercising and professing to have that special skill. A man need not*

possess the highest expert skill; it is well-established law that it is sufficient if he exercises the ordinary skill of an ordinary competent man exercising that particular art.[18]

McNair specifically asked the jury to consider whether this principle applied to the question of adequate information:

when the defendants adopted the practice they did (namely, the practice of saying very little and waiting for questions from the patient), they were falling below a proper standard of competent professional opinion on the question of whether or not it is right to warn.[18]

McNair considered it unlikely that John Bolam would have refused treatment even if he had been aware of the risk. This again demonstrates the difficulty that plaintiffs can experience when seeking to prove negligence. The jury held that the clinical practice at Friern Hospital was consistent with 'competent professional opinion'. On this basis, judgement was for the defendants.

This case established the principle that professionals were to be judged against the standards of their peers. Until recently, the range of acceptable practice was seldom clearly defined, and the scope of the duty of disclosure of risk was left in the hands of the medical profession. In 1981, in *Chatterton v Gerson and another*,[19] Bristow J did not believe that Elizabeth Chatterton, who was desperate because of pain, would have refused treatment if she had been told about its side-effects. Her action failed in both negligence and trespass. In Bristow J's view:

Once the patient is informed in broad terms of the nature of the procedure . . . and gives her consent, that consent is real, and the cause of the action on which to base a claim for failure to go into risks and implications is negligence, not trespass.[19]

The standard of disclosure adopted by Bristow J for a claim in negligence was that of *Bolam v Friern Hospital Management Committee*,[18] and that a clinician 'ought to warn of what may happen by misfortune . . . if there is a real risk of misfortune in the procedure'.[19]

In practice, the problem lies with defining what is a real risk of misfortune. Is it a risk of 1 in 10 or 1 in 1000? Or is it a risk of specific concern to an individual patient? Amy Sidaway had suffered recurrent pain in her neck, right shoulder and arm. A senior neurosurgeon, Murray Faulkner, advised her to undergo surgery, which carried a 1–2% risk of damage to the spinal nerve roots, but failed to warn her of the lesser but more serious risk of damage to the spinal cord. In her claim for damages she relied 'on the alleged failure of the surgeon to disclose or explain to her the risks inherent in, or special to, the operation which he had advised'.[20]

The judge recognised that omission of detailed information about uncommon risks was standard practice at the time, and so in keeping with the principles identified in *Bolam v Friern Hospital Management Committee*.[18] The judge dismissed her claim, but acknowledged that if the nature of the operation had been fully explained to her, she would not have agreed to it. The case was appealed.

In his summary, Lord Diplock pointed out that the case concerned:

> *volunteering unsought information about risks . . . To decide what risks the existence of which a patient should be voluntarily warned . . . is as much an exercise of professional skill and judgement as any other part of the doctor's comprehensive duty of care to the individual patient . . . The* Bolam *test should be applied.*[21]

The House of Lords' decision placed the responsibility for discussing risk on doctors. However, only the vaguest of guidelines about the magnitude of risk that must be discussed can be extracted from the judgement. Lord Bridge confirmed the role of clinicians, but also recognised the fact that some risks were so great that any prudent doctor would disclose them.

> *I am of the opinion that the judge might in certain circumstances come to the conclusion that disclosure of a particular risk was so obviously necessary to an informed choice on the part of the patient that no reasonably prudent man would fail to make it. The kind of case I have in mind would be an operation involving a substantial risk of grave adverse consequences, as, for example, the 10% risk of a stroke from the operation which was the subject of the Canadian Case Reibl v Hughes, 114 DELR (3d) 1.*[22]

The view of Dunn LJ as expressed in the Court of Appeal was accepted: 'The doctrine of informed consent has no place in English law'.[23]

Although Lord Scarman agreed that the plaintiff's appeal should be dismissed on its facts, he delivered a dissenting speech on the aspect of disclosure of risk:

> *In a medical negligence case where the issue is the advice and information given to the patient as to the treatment proposed, the available options, and the risk, the court is concerned primarily with a patient's right . . . for the proper implementation of the right requires that the doctor be under a duty to inform his patient of the material risks inherent in the*

> treatment . . . *The law can . . . do the next best thing and require the court to answer the question, what would a reasonably prudent patient think significant if in the situation of this patient?*[24]

The view held was that there was no doctrine in English law that patients were entitled to know everything, just as there was no concept that doctors were entitled to decide everything. The outcome of this case was that the information given to patients before surgery was not a matter of meeting objective criteria, but a matter for doctors to decide. If they blundered, damages would be payable.

However, public concerns that have come to the fore in the 1990s in association with the Bristol Inquiry have placed the Department of Health's view alongside that of Lord Scarman. The disclosure of detailed information about risks of procedures and competence of practitioners is likely to become standard practice, driven forward by employers, the NHS Litigation Authority and the Clinical Negligence Scheme for Trusts.

The impact of *Sidaway v Bethlehem Royal Hospital Governors* can be seen in the Department of Health's document, *Reference Guide to Consent for Examination or Treatment*, which states:

> that it was open to the courts to decide that information about a particular risk was so obviously necessary that it would be negligent not to provide it, even if a 'responsible body' of medical opinion would not have done so.[25]

Such views about limited provision of information were confirmed in *Blyth v Bloomsbury Health Authority*.[26] The case revolved around the fact that the plaintiff had specifically asked about potential side-effects of the contraceptive drug, Provera. Although the Court of Appeal held that it was a doctor's duty to answer questions, the detail would depend upon circumstances and need not be comprehensive. Answers would be judged in the light of responsible medical opinion and practice at the time. Although *Smith v Tunbridge Wells Health Authority*[27] may appear to run contrary to these decisions, it does in fact support them. According to Mr Justice Morland:

> *The issue in the case was whether Mr Cook was under a duty to explain to the plaintiff the particular risks of impotence and bladder dysfunction which can arise through mishap in a Wells operation; also if Mr Cook had that duty whether he discharged it. The further issue is whether the plaintiff would have declined the Wells operation if the explanation of the risk had been given.*[28]

The plaintiff's submission was that 'the consent to the operation was not informed consent, and therefore not consent'.[28]

This view was supported by the fact that a responsible body of medical opinion, including Mr Cook, regarded an explanation of the risks of impotence to a young sexually active man as mandatory. In reviewing the Sidaway case, Morland J drew attention to the comments of Lord Templeman: 'A patient may make an unbalanced judgement because he is deprived of adequate information'.[29]

In this case, the need to disclose the possible complication of impotence in a young man 'was so obviously necessary that it would be negligent not to provide it'.[25]

However, Margaret Puxon, in writing a commentary on the case, made the following observations:

> This case is a warning to doctors that they cannot afford to rely on even the highest authority in their specialty as to the extent of the information that they should give when obtaining consent: the only guidance they get from this case is that they must act 'reasonably', that is in a manner which a court would find 'reasonable'. And how are they to know what the court would find 'reasonable'? Perhaps we are back to the subjective test, but not only the test of what the particular patient requires, but what a hypothetical judge may require if ever a court is asked to adjudicate. Indeed, the doctor's lot is not an entirely happy one.[30]

Support for Margaret Puxon's view about the role of authorities within a specialty comes from *Bolitho v City & Hackney Health Authority*.[31] During this case, expert witnesses disagreed about the way in which they would have cared for Patrick Bolitho. Lord Browne-Wilkinson said:

> the court is not bound to hold that a defendant doctor escapes liability for negligent treatment or diagnosis just because he leads evidence from a number of medical experts who are genuinely of opinion that the defendant's treatment or diagnosis accorded with sound medical practice.[32]

The future significance of *Bolitho v City & Hackney Health Authority* lies with the possibility that similar thinking will be applied to the disclosure of risk. The Department of Health and many professional specialist bodies are moving towards a standard where detailed discussion of risks, complications and alternative forms of treatment will become standard practice. The courts may not see the contrary view, although held by some experts, as reasoned or responsible.

> *The use of these adjectives – responsible, reasonable and respectable – all show that the court has to be satisfied that the exponents of the body of opinion relied upon can demonstrate that such opinion has a logical basis.*[32]

Thus a failure to provide adequately detailed information about an intervention may come to be regarded as negligent.

The introduction into domestic English law of the provisions of the European Convention on Human Rights is likely to affect judgements on issues related to consent, as it is a human rights issue with respect for bodily integrity and privacy central to the convention.[33] In his editorial, McCall Smith summarised the current position in the following words:

> *Now, in cases such as Bolitho and Pearce, the courts have said that they will depart from the professional practice approach if they see fit, the ultimate legal test being what the court itself thinks was a reasonable amount of information to give the patient. But how, one might wonder, is a doctor going to be able to reach that decision? Doctors cannot guess what the courts are going to say. All they can do is ask themselves, is this what my professional peers would consider the proper thing to do? This leaves an element of doubt, which no amount of guidance from the Department of Health will ever be able to dispel.*[33]

While there is no clear guidance as to what is a reasonable risk, clinicians will continue to feel vulnerable, and there will be wide discrepancies in the degree of disclosure between various units. In a later section I shall review the introduction of statute law in some jurisdictions, which is concerned with disclosure in an attempt to overcome this difficulty.

Disclosure of risk and patients' questions

In *Pearce v United Bristol Healthcare NHS Trust*,[34] an obstetrician failed to tell Mrs Pearce of the 0.1% to 0.2% risk of a stillbirth. Although the Court of Appeal recognised that if a patient asked about risks a doctor was obliged to give an honest answer, the degree of disclosure was a matter of clinical judgement. In this case the Court felt that Mrs Pearce's obstetrician had been right to shield her from this information, because of her distress at the time.

The definition of what is a significant risk is problematic, and Lord Woolf stated that:

*In the Sidaway case Lord Bridge . . . refers to a 'significant risk'
as being a risk of something in the region of 10 per cent. When
one refers to a 'significant risk', it is not possible to talk in
percentages, but I note, and it may be purely coincidental . . .
that one of the expert doctors . . . gave the following answer . . .
if the risk, however, was of the order of 10 per cent, for
instance, then of course it would be my duty to warn against
such a level of risk.*[35]

Clearly the Court was concerned to say that it was not possible to express
'significant risk' in percentage terms. Indeed, what is a significant risk
for one patient may not be so for another, and this will be independent of
frequency of occurrence.[36] The need to provide adequate information
then becomes a balance between the patient's wish for autonomy and
the clinician's paternalistic concerns about adverse effects on the
patient's welfare.

The Australian case of *Rogers v Whitaker*[36] concerned the failure of an
ophthalmic surgeon to warn Maree Whitaker of the risk of blindness in a
good eye following surgery to improve the sight of her damaged other
eye. Central to this case was the fact that Maree Whitaker wanted to
know the risks of the procedure and kept on questioning Christopher
Rogers about them. Campbell J accepted that:

*a doctor has a duty to warn a patient of a material risk
inherent in the proposed treatment . . . in the circumstances
of the particular case, a reasonable person in the patient's
position, if warned of the risk, would be likely to attach
significance to it or if the medical practitioner is or should
reasonably be aware that the particular patient, if warned of
the risk, would be likely to attach significance to it.*[36]

Although this case is often quoted as suggesting that doctors should
warn patients of risks as low as 1 in 14 000, this is not the case. The
ceiling is not defined in numerical terms. Rather it is a risk, which is
'real and foreseeable'. Indeed, in Australia the situation is that it:

*is for the courts to adjudicate on what is the appropriate
standard of care after giving weight to 'the paramount consideration that a person is entitled to make his own decisions
about his life'.*[37]

This case can be persuasive within England and Wales, and clearly
persistent questioning by a patient should be answered truthfully.
During the consent process the patient needs to be encouraged to

reveal their anxieties and ask any questions which might be of concern to them.

The intelligibility of information

In *Smith v Tunbridge Wells Health Authority*,[30] Morland J made the important point that:

> The doctor, when warning of the risks, must take reasonable care to ensure that his explanation of the risks is intelligible to his particular patient. The doctor should use language [that is] simple but not misleading.[30]

In *Pearce v United Bristol Healthcare NHS Trust*,[35] Lord Woolf expressed similar views about providing information on risk: 'The doctor . . . has to take into account . . . the ability of the patient to comprehend what he has to say to him or her'.[35]

In *Gillian Karen Carver v Hammersmith & Queen Charlotte's Special Health Authority*,[38] a senior house officer (SHO) who discussed the Bart's test failed to explain that it was only a screening test and, unlike amniocentesis, not diagnostic. Ms Carver had a child with Down's syndrome, and the health authority was found liable in negligence. Nelson J held that the SHO's:

> explanation of the test generally was not given in such terms as could reasonably have brought home to her the fact that the test was not diagnostic. As a result, the claimant came away from the consultation with the doctor with the clear, albeit mistaken, view that the Bart's test would determine whether or not she had a handicapped child.[38]

Clearly the quality of information and the way in which it is understood are critical. The fact that the client was told about the test was inadequate. She needed sufficient information to enable her to make a balanced decision, and the clinical judgement of the SHO should have taken into account Gillian Carver's determination to avoid having a handicapped child.

A similar concern exists with regard to the ability of a patient to understand English, as was seen in the Canadian case of *Reibl v Hughes*:[39]

> It must have been obvious to the defendant that the plaintiff had some difficulty with the English language and

that he should, therefore, have made certain that he was understood.[39]

Although this has not yet been an issue in medical cases, it has been of importance in other situations.[40,41] Clearly there needs to be provision of accurate translation when seeking consent from a patient for whom English is not their first language.

Disclosure in other jurisdictions

Interest in the degree of disclosure of risk and alternatives in the USA followed on from *Cooper v Roberts*.[42] Irene Cooper brought an action against her physicians because they had perforated her stomach during an examination of her hiatus hernia with a flexible gastroscope. The court held that in order for there to:

> have been an 'informed and knowledgeable' consent, the physician should have advised the patient of the consequences of the operation as well as the alternative possibilities.[42]

The US court had rejected any suggestion that physicians could keep secret the possible complications of surgery. It rejected a professional standard of disclosure, rather choosing a 'reasonable person standard'.[8] The court's decision was jointly based on the views that:

> To hold otherwise would permit the medical profession to determine its own responsibilities to the patients in a matter of considerable public interest.[42]

and:

> As the patient must bear the expense, pain and suffering of any injury from medical treatment, his right to know all material facts pertaining to the proposed treatment cannot depend upon the self-imposed standards of the medical profession.[42]

Such views reflect many of the ideas currently expressed in the UK. The failure of the General Medical Council to reassure the public adequately that they are appropriately monitoring the medical profession has led to calls for radical changes in the ways in which the healthcare professions are regulated.

A year later, in *Canterbury v Spence*,[43] Robinson J confirmed the need for statute law to regulate disclosure in the USA. In this case, a

19-year-old man had agreed to a laminectomy without being warned of the risk of paralysis.

> *Respect for the patient's right of self-determination on particular therapy demands a standard set by law for physicians, rather than one which physicians may or may not impose on themselves.*[43]

This is the 'prudent patient' test for the need for information. However, Robinson J still argued for some therapeutic privilege to be left with clinicians. In the 1980s, two Canadian cases[39,44] followed this American lead and recognised that:

> *In obtaining the consent of a patient for the performance upon him of a surgical operation, a surgeon, generally, should answer any specific questions posed by the patient as to the risks involved, and should, without being questioned, disclose to him the nature of the proposed operation, its gravity, any material risks and any special or unusual risks.*[44]

From these cases and *Arndt v Smith*,[45] Canada has developed a 'reasonable patient' test, which has objective elements rather than just subjective ones. It:

> *must take into consideration any 'particular concerns' of the patient and any 'special considerations affecting the particular patient' in determining whether the patient would have refused treatment if given all the information about the possible risks. The 'reasonable person' who sets the standard for the objective test must be taken to possess the patient's reasonable beliefs, fears, desires and expectations.*[45]

The benefits of this test are that it is balanced, favouring neither the plaintiff nor the clinician. As in the USA, some Canadian states have embodied these concepts within statute law. In contrast to the situation in England and Wales, when this happens both patients and clinicians have a clearer understanding of the nature of the information that must be exchanged as part of the consent process.

Despite the outcome in the Australian case of *Rogers v Whitaker*,[36] the judges criticised the US concepts of 'a patient's right of self-determination' and 'informed consent'. They felt that a failure to disclose detailed risks of a procedure was negligent rather than related to the offence of battery. The acceptance of a 'reasonable person' test in Australia still means that such decisions can be subjective. In *Rosenberg v Percival*,[16] the court recognised that unlike the USA and Canada,

'Australia has rejected the objective test of causation in favour of a subjective one'.[16]

Australia is concerned whether 'this patient' would have undergone a procedure, and what a 'reasonable person' would have done is not conclusive. The decision as to what 'this patient' would have done depends on his or her credibility. Indeed, Gummow J recognised the difficulties in these circumstances of defining what level of risk should be discussed with a patient, and he returned to the Bolam principle when he wrote: 'these factors are to be considered from the point of view of what a reasonable medical practitioner . . . ought to have foreseen at the time'.[16]

When disclosure of risk depends on what individual patients might want to know, guidelines for clinicians need to ensure that patients' anxieties are identified during the consent process. Australia has resisted any movement to formalise consent into any statute, but rather has endorsed the issuing of *General Guidelines for Medical Practitioners on Providing Information to Patients* by the National Health and Medical Research Council of Australia in 1993.[46] These are very similar to the more recent guidelines issued in 2001 by the Department of Health in England and Wales.[25]

References

1 Hawkins C (1985) *Mishap or Malpractice?* Blackwell Scientific Publications, Oxford.

2 *Slater v Baker and Stapleton* [1767] 8 Geo 111 860–63.

3 *Slater v Baker and Stapleton* [1767] 8 Geo 111 860 at 860 (section 359).

4 *Slater v Baker and Stapleton* [1767] 8 Geo 111 860 at 862 (section 361).

5 *Slater v Baker and Stapleton* [1767] 8 Geo 111 860 at 861 (section 360).

6 *Schloendorff v The Society of the New York Hospitals* [1914] 211 NY 125, 105 NE 92.

7 Katz J (1984) *The Silent World of Doctor and Patient.* The Free Press, New York.

8 Faden RR, Beauchamp TL and King NMP (1986) *A History of Informed Consent.* Oxford University Press, New York.

9 *Salgo v Leland Stanford Junior University Board of Trustees* [1957] 317 P.2d 170, 181 (Cal. Dist. Ct. App. 1957).

10 *Breen v Baker* [1956] *The Times* 27 January.

11 NHS Management Executive (1990) *A Guide to Consent for Examination or Treatment.* NHS Management Executive, London.

12 *Christine Williamson v East London and the City Health Authority and Others* [1998] 1 Lloyd's Rep Med 6: [1998] 41 BMLR 85.

13 *Natanson v Kline* [1960] 350 P.2d 1093 (Kan. 1960).

14 Smith HW (1946) Therapeutic privilege to withhold specific diagnosis from patient sick with serious or fatal illness. *Tennessee Law Rev.* **19**: 349f.

15 *Hills v Potter & Anor* [1984] 1 WLR 641: [1983] 3 AER 716.

16 *Rosenberg v Percival* [2001] 178 ALR 577.

17 *Walsh v Irish Family Planning Services* [1992] 1 IR 496.

18 *Bolam v Friern Hospital Management Committee* [1957] 1 WLR 582–94.

19 *Chatterton v Gerson and another* [1981] 1 QB 432–45.

20 *Sidaway v Bethlehem Royal Hospital Governors* [1984] 1 All ER 1018, CA, [1985] 1 BMLR 132.

21 *Sidaway v Bethlehem Royal Hospital Governors* [1985] AC 871 at 895.

22 *Sidaway v Bethlehem Royal Hospital Governors* [1985] AC 871 at 899.

23 *Sidaway v Bethlehem Royal Hospital Governors* [1984] 1 QB 493 at 517.

24 *Sidaway v Bethlehem Royal Hospital Governors* [1985] AC 871 at 888.

25 Department of Health (2001) *Reference Guide to Consent for Examination or Treatment*. Department of Health, London.

26 *Blyth v Bloomsbury Health Authority* [1987] ILR 9/2/1987: TLR 11/2/1987: [1993] 4 Med LR 151.

27 *Smith v Tunbridge Wells Health Authority* [1994] 5 Med LR 334.

28 *Smith v Tunbridge Wells Health Authority* [1994] 5 Med LR 334 at 335.

29 *Smith v Tunbridge Wells Health Authority* [1994] 5 Med LR 334 at 337.

30 *Smith v Tunbridge Wells Health Authority* [1994] 5 Med LR 334 at 342.

31 *Bolitho v City & Hackney Health Authority* [1997] LTL 14/11/1997: TLR 27/11/97: [1997] 3 WLR 1151: [1997] 4 All ER 771: [1998] 1 Lloyd's Rep Med 26: [1998] 39 BMLR 1: [1998] 1 PNLR 1: [1993] 4 Med LR 381.

32 *Bolitho v City & Hackney Health Authority* [1997] 4 All ER 771, HL (quoted in Stauch M, Wheat K and Tingle J (1998) *Sourcebook on Medical Law*. Cavendish Publishing Ltd, London).

33 McCall Smith A (2001) Obtaining consent for examination and treatment. *BMJ.* **322**: 810–11.

34 *Pearce v United Bristol Healthcare NHS Trust* [1999] 48 BMLR 118.

35 *Pearce v United Bristol Healthcare NHS Trust* [1998] EWCA Civ 865 (20 May 1998) at 23 (from www.bailii.org).

36 *Rogers v Whitaker* [1992] 175 CLR 479, 109 ALR 625, 16 BMLR 148.

37 *Rogers v Whitaker* [1992] 109 ALR 625, p. 6 of *Australian Law Reports* (Reed International Books, Australia Pty Ltd).

38 *Gillian Karen Carver v Hammersmith & Queen Charlotte's Special Health*

Authority [2000] QBD (Nelson J0 25/2/2000), LTL 10/4/2000 (unreported elsewhere).

39 *Reibl v Hughes* [1980] 2 SCR 880, 114 DLR (93d) 1 14CCLT 1, Can SC (quoted in http://qsilver.queensu.ca/law/restrict/peppin. . . . . ./Reibl).

40 *Kunnath v The State* [1993] 4 All ER 30: [1993] 1 WLR 1315: [1993] 98 CAR 455: Guardian 20/8/93 [1993] 137 SJ(LB) 195: [1993] 143 NLJ 1332: TLR 30/7/93.

41 *Hamid Dedsahti Haghighat v (1) Abdul Razzak Mohammed Rakim Baksh (2) James Hebblethwaite and Baksh (a firm) (3) Djaved Sepjani (4) Chatwani and Co (a firm): Solicitors' Indemnity Fund (substituted for TSB Bank plc) v (1) Djaved Sepjani (2) Hamid Dedsahti Haghighat* [1999] LTL 27/10/99 Extempore (unreported elsewhere). Document no. C8400534.

42 *Cooper v Roberts* [1971] 220 Pa. Super. 260, 286 A.2d 647.

43 *Canterbury v Spence* [1972] 464 F. 2d 772, 784 (D.C. Cir. 1972).

44 *Hopp v Lepp* [1980] 2 SCR 192.

45 *Arndt v Smith* [1997] 2 SCR 5 (quoted in http://canlii.org/ca/cas/scc/1997/1997scc65.html).

46 National Health and Medical Research Council of Australia (1993) *General Guidelines for Medical Practitioners on Providing Information to Patients.* National Health and Medical Research Council of Australia, Canberra.

Chapter 4

Consent to investigation and treatment: the views of Government and professional organisations

Introduction

In this chapter, the impact of policy and medical thinking on consent practice will be considered. This is likely to form the basis on which the courts will assess contemporary practice. Governmental bodies and professional organisations concerned with healthcare are keen to promote evidence-based practice and so to establish uniform standards to be met by clinicians. *Bolam v Friern Hospital Management Committee* stated that: 'it is well-established law that it is sufficient if he exercises the ordinary skill of an ordinary competent man exercising that particular art'.[1]

Competent clinicians will be expected to follow national guidelines. Although there will be experts who may disagree with the standards of investigation and treatment advocated by these bodies, *Bolitho v City & Hackney Health Authority* has made it clear that 'there are cases where, despite a body of professional opinion sanctioning the defendant's conduct, the defendant can properly be held liable for negligence'.[2]

Such an approach may well be applied to standards of disclosure as well as therapy. During the past decade a range of organisations have taken an interest in the consent process. The common theme is that informed consent is the minimum standard to which clinicians should practise, and this has arisen because of legal demands. The irony of this position is that this view is not held by the courts. However, as with the *amicus* brief submitted by the American College of Surgeons in *Salgo v Leland Stanford Junior University Board of Trustees*,[3] judges might come to view it as ordinary practice under the Bolam rule.

The role of the Department of Health

An interesting question arises with regard to the role of the Department of Health and the Secretary of State for Health in the consent process. Do they owe a duty of care to the patients? And if so, could that include the provision of adequate information about procedures, including their risks and complications? In addition, the Department holds information on local and individual performance. Should this be made available to the public? Clearly, this type of information will be important when patients are given the opportunity to select their surgeon.

Section 3 of the National Health Service Act 1977 gives wide discretion to the Secretary of State, and it is unlikely that any action against the minister would be successful. In *Re HIV Haemophiliac Litigation*,[4] Bingham LJ drew an analogy with *Hill v Chief Constable of Yorkshire*:[5]

> *Strong reasons of public policy (or justice and reasonableness) for not holding a minister and department exercising public functions for the benefit of the community as a whole to owe a duty of care towards individual members of the public.*[4]

Although the senior administration of the Department of Health seem to be safe from litigation, the recent issue of its *Reference Guide to Consent for Examination or Treatment* recognises that:

> *Although this Guidance focuses primarily on the legal position, it will also indicate where regulatory bodies have set out more stringent requirements. It should be noted that the legal requirements in negligence cases have historically been based on the standards set by the professions for their members, and hence where standards required by professional bodies are rising, it is likely that the legal standards will rise accordingly.*[6]

The Secretary of State for Health, Alan Milburn, distanced himself from the paternalism which he believes characterises the medical profession, and on 30 January 2001 he said that fundamental changes are needed in the laws governing patients' consent:

> *Above all else, for trust to thrive there has to be informed consent. Not a tick in the box consent regime but consent based on discussion and dialogue, where consent is actively sought and positively given . . . It has to take patients into its confidence.*[7]

Although such views do not carry any legal weight, there is growing commitment in the Department of Health to greater information and to the concept of informed consent. Its commitment to the provision of more information so that patients can arrive at a balanced decision means that the standard of care which is being set by the Department of Health is one of 'informed consent'.

The development of clinical guidelines on consent

During the past decade there has been considerable movement towards formulation of best clinical practice in the form of guidelines. Such guidelines have been directed at consent processes, investigative techniques and clinical treatment. Their role is to ensure widespread dissemination of good practice, and as such to codify the principles identified in *Bolam v Friern Hospital Management Committee.*[1] Their legal status has been reviewed in *Caroline Smith v National Health Service Litigation Authority.*[8] At the time of the claimant's birth in 1973 it was common practice to test newborn children for congenital dislocation of the hip. This practice followed the advice prepared by the Standing Medical Advisory Committee in a set of what would later be called 'guidelines'. Andrew Smith J held that: 'Whilst the guidelines were not to be interpreted as a statute, they were evidence of good medical practice at the time the claimant was born'.[8]

This still represents the clinical status of guidelines. Guidelines represent correct treatment, not the highest standards of care, as some believe. Their introduction has paralleled the emergence of greater patient autonomy. Aspects of this approach are enshrined in the Human Rights Act 1998 and in the modernisation of the NHS. Harpwood has written:

> *Early results from the second national NHS survey of patients confirm patients want to be better informed about their treatment so that they can be more involved in making decisions about their own care . . . This suggests that in future the question of patient autonomy may be a consideration for judges when they decide cases concerning information provision and consent to treatment.*[9]

Together with others,[10] she has suggested that in the British legal system 'progress towards respecting values such as autonomy has been leaden footed, and behind developments in other jurisdictions'.[9]

It is likely that doctors will be required by their employers and patients to comply with national and local guidelines on consent and management issues.

The Patient's Charter

A Conservative Government introduced The Patient's Charter in an attempt to make the National Health Service more accountable to its clients – the patients. It was an attempt to state in clear and simple language what patients might expect from their carers. It claimed that all patients have a right:

> to be given a clear explanation of any treatment proposed, including any risks and alternatives, before [they] decide whether [they] will agree to the treatment.[11]

It is debatable whether the law in England and Wales gives patients such a right. However, the Charter was the first Government document to encourage clinicians and patients to consider that the minimum standard of care required was based around the concept of informed consent.

The Department of Health's *Reference Guide to Consent for Examination or Treatment*

In 2001, the Department of Health published guidelines on consent. Section 1.5 deals with the specific question of whether the patient has received sufficient information:

> Although informing patients of the nature and purpose of procedures enables valid consent to be given so far as any claim of battery is concerned, this is not sufficient to fulfil the legal duty of care to the patient. Failure to provide other relevant information may render the professional liable to an action for negligence if a patient subsequently suffers harm as a result of the treatment received.[6]

Advice given in the guidelines includes the following:

> *Inform the patient of any 'material' or 'significant' risks in the proposed treatment, any alternatives to it, and the risks incurred by doing nothing.*[6]

> *The mere fact that the patient might become upset by hearing the information, or might refuse treatment, is not sufficient to act as justification [for withholding information].*[6]

However, the document recognises in section 5.2 that:

> *It is now clear that the courts will be the final arbiter of what constitutes responsible practice, although the standards set by the health professions for their members will still be influential.*[6]

In parallel with the publication of the *Reference Guide*, the Department of Health produced *Consent. What You Have a Right to Expect. A Guide for Adults.*[12] This explains to the public how consent should operate in NHS hospitals in England and Wales. The website also points patients in the direction of organisations that are able to offer further support with regard to consent-related issues. Among these is Patient Concern. This organisation produces a series of leaflets, including one on 'How to survive surgery',[13] which states that:

> *Every operation or medical treatment is a balance of risks and benefits so, before you agree to any procedure, your doctor must explain these risks and benefits so that you can give informed consent.*[13]

The general tone of information and advice from the Department of Health is that patients should expect to be fully informed about procedures, and the concept of 'informed consent' is accepted as good practice within NHS hospitals. Indeed it is more than good practice – it is the standard by which all clinicians should work. These new standards are reflected in the new 'consent' form or 'patient agreement to investigation, treatment or operation'. A detailed series of consent forms are now available. In these new forms clinicians are expected to:

> *Describe . . . what is proposed in everyday language, including (a) the aim of the procedure, (b) serious or frequently occurring risks, (c) any alternative treatments which may be available and (d) what the patient will experience afterwards, including common side-effects. Where applicable this can be done over several visits.*[14]

Clinicians will also have to sign the following statement: 'I also confirm that I have the necessary competence to provide this information'.[14]

This will restrict consent to someone who is able to undertake the procedure or who has received specific training about methods, alternatives and complications, although they are personally unable to do it.

If there are language problems, the following statement needs to be signed:

> *If interpreter is present*: I have interpreted the information . . .
> to the patient to the best of my ability and in terms which I
> believe he/she can understand.[14]

In the latest guidelines issued on the Department's website, special attention is given to the need to ensure that elderly patients have a proper understanding of the information that they have received during the consent process.[14]

The NHS Litigation Authority

In 1995, the National Health Service Litigation Authority was created as a Special Health Authority under section 21(3) of the National Health Service and Community Care Act 1990. An early function was the administration of the Clinical Negligence Scheme for Trusts. Standard 5 of the Scheme deals with 'Advice and Consent' and requires:

> *Appropriate information is provided to patients on the risks*
> *and benefits of the proposed treatment or investigation, and*
> *the alternatives available, before a signature on a consent*
> *form is sought . . .*
> *Doctors must ensure . . . they have established:*
> * *what the patient wants to know*
> * *what the patient ought to know*
> * *that the patient understands the information which has*
>   *been given*
> * *that the patient consents to the treatment.*[15]

Trusts can comply with this standard at one of three levels. At level 3 the scheme requires 'the trust to be actively helping patients to obtain further information about their conditions and proposed treatment if they so wish'.[15]

This could include self-help groups, internet addresses and an information centre within the hospital. The standards being set for clinical practice within England and Wales are those in which patients are extensively educated about their disease and its management. The Bolam and Bolitho principles will in the future operate in an environment where 'informed consent' is seen as the accepted standard of good clinical care. The interesting question which arises from the work of the Authority and the Scheme is what the motivating factor was for these developments. The answer may well be that it was the perception that this was the level of information giving required to limit litigation!

Methods of assessing comprehension and ability to use information in the elderly can be summarised as follows.

- Explore the patient's ability to paraphrase what has been said (repeating and rewording explanations as necessary).
- Explore whether the patient is able to compare alternatives.
- Explore whether the patient has any thoughts about possible consequences other than those which you have disclosed.
- Explore whether the patient applies the information to their own case.

Some patients may therefore have the capacity to consent to some interventions but not to others. For example, people suffering from the early stages of dementia would probably still have the capacity to make many straightforward decisions about their own care (e.g. washing or bathing, or whether or not to have an operation to correct a hernia), but might lack the capacity to make very complex decisions.[16]

The role of the General Medical Council and the Nursing and Midwifery Council (formerly the United Kingdom Central Council for Nursing, Midwifery and Health Visiting)

In *Good Medical Practice 2001*,[17] the guidance for obtaining consent is summarised as follows:

> You must respect the rights of patients to be fully involved in decisions about their care. Wherever possible you must be satisfied, before you provide treatment or investigate a patient's condition, that the patient has understood what is proposed, and why, any significant risks or side-effects associated with it, and has given consent.[17]

Detailed guidelines are laid out in *Seeking Patients' Consent: the ethical considerations*.[18] The discussion of risks forms an important part of this advice, and it calls on doctors to ask patients:

> *whether they have any concerns about the treatment or the*
> *risks it may involve . . . Ask patients whether they have*
> *understood the information and whether they would like*
> *more before making a decision.*[18]

The General Medical Council's document sees consent as a process. It encourages doctors to allow patients time to reflect, to provide information in manageable amounts and to use up-to-date written material and visual and other aids. It deals specifically with language and communication difficulties:

> *Make arrangements . . . to meet particular language and*
> *communication needs . . . through translations, independent*
> *interpreters, signers or the patient's representative.*[18]

The General Medical Council recognises the autonomy of patients and believes that they should be able 'to exercise their right to make informed decisions about their care'.[18]

It also believes, with little foundation, that this right to an informed choice is 'protected in law'.[18]

The UKCC's *Guidelines for Professional Practice*[19] tell nurses of similar responsibilities:

> *It is not safe to assume that the patient or client has enough*
> *knowledge, even about basic treatment, for them to make an*
> *informed choice without an explanation.*[19]

The role of a specialist society

In 1999 the British Society of Gastroenterology published *Guidelines for Informed Consent for Endoscopic Procedures*. Its opening statement is as follows: 'Informed consent is a cornerstone of good medical practice'.[20]

Interestingly, the authors believed that 'over the last 30 years informed consent for a medical procedure has been transformed from an ethical concept to a legal requirement'.[20]

The authors had taken advice from a QC during the drafting of the document. Such views are commonly held by specialist practitioners. The British Society of Gastroenterology is representative of the views of many similar societies and reflects the advice given to their members.

All of these groups, from the Department of Health to specialist societies, now recognise informed consent as required practice. It cannot be long before the courts recognise this, too. The recommendations from the inquiry into cardiac surgery in Bristol can only strengthen the position of those who advocate informed consent.

The Bristol Royal Infirmary Inquiry

The tragic death of so many children who were receiving complex heart surgery at Bristol Royal Infirmary led to a public inquiry which challenged most aspects of traditional care. It called for greater empowerment of patients, and stated that one of the principal ways of achieving this 'is to ensure that they [patients] have the necessary information to allow them to understand and participate in their care to the extent desired'.[21]

The concept of a paternalistic and benevolent doctor would be swept away. The current legal stance of the doctor making a clinical decision as to the extent of information a patient should receive is challenged. The Inquiry felt that:

> the issue is no longer whether to inform a patient, but how to do so effectively . . . We believe that healthcare professionals have a duty to empower patients, and providing information is one means of empowerment. We accept that each patient is different and may wish for varying amounts of information at various times, with the constant ability to say 'enough'. But this fact does not serve as a reason for not setting out on the information journey.[21]

In order to achieve these objectives, the Inquiry recognised that in practice:

> patients . . . should always be given the opportunity and time to ask questions about what they are told, to seek clarification, and to ask for more information.[21]

Under these circumstances, the Inquiry believed that 'consent should be seen as an ongoing process of informed decision-making'.[21]

The Inquiry gave unreserved support to the need for healthcare professionals to be open and honest with patients and to provide them with comprehensive information about examinations, investigations and treatments. The purpose of this information is to empower the patient to make a choice – this is informed consent. The impact of the Inquiry on the management of healthcare in England and Wales will be profound. The standards that it has called for are already being put in place as a result of the Clinical Negligence Scheme for Trusts and the impact of the General Medical Council and UKCC guidance. However, none of these have the impact of statute or case law, except through the Bolam and Bolitho principles. The Human Rights Act 1998 states that:

> *failure to act in a way that is compatible with human rights as stated in the Convention may lead to a legal claim . . . and that they can seek remedies from the courts in the UK.*[9]

Cases where the patient's consent is in question could involve human rights issues under Article 3 of the Convention, and this could open up a new field of legal remedy.

Although judges in England and Wales may have rejected the transatlantic concept of informed consent, it seems unlikely that such a view will stand when the accepted standard of practice requires that clinicians practise this doctrine. Through Bolam and Bolitho, informed consent will be seen as the form of practice which an average competent doctor exercises on a daily basis. The problems that remain include which risks clinicians must disclose. However, there may be a transatlantic solution to this.

Current situation in the USA

Informed consent led to significant litigation in the USA. It was characterised by the problem of what level of risk should be routinely disclosed, as well as specific risks of concern to particular patients. As a result, some states have passed legislation which requires that such risks as brain damage, paralysis or loss of function of an organ and disfiguring scars must always be disclosed, even when those risks are very small.[22] This approach depersonalises the relationship between the doctor and the patient. In some states there is no mandatory requirement to disclose any other risks in order to obtain informed consent. However, in 1989 the Louisiana Supreme Court in *Hondroulis v Schumacher* ruled that 'loss of function of an organ'[23] was too generic, and that doctors needed to be more specific. The surgeon had failed to mention specifically that loss of bladder function could be a complication of a lumbar laminectomy. This led to doctors listing many potential risks when seeking consent. In 1990, the Louisiana legislature passed the Uniform Consent Law and created a Medical Disclosure Panel (R.S. 40: 1299.40E).[22] The purpose of the panel is to define which risks must be disclosed for any given procedure. The panel consists of six doctors, a dentist and four attorneys, and it meets bimonthly. It is developing a list of risks for all procedures.

Such a development addresses the thorny question of how much to disclose, and removes it both from the individual clinician and from the court. The format of the disclosure is as follows:

> *in writing, signed by the patient or a person authorised to give the consent and by a competent witness, and if the written consent specifically states, in such terms and language that a layman would be expected to understand, the risks and hazards that are involved in the medical care or surgical procedure in the form and to the degree required by the panel.*[22]

Provided that Louisiana clinicians comply, this will be strong evidence against accusations of negligence linked to a failure to obtain informed consent.

The precedent for a Medical Disclosure Panel was set in 1979 by the Medical Liability and Insurance Improvement Act of Texas.[24] In this Act, hysterectomy was seen as a specific problem area (section 6.08), and the need was recognised that information about the procedure and its risks:

> *shall be available in English, Spanish, and any other language the panel considers appropriate. The information shall be presented in a manner understandable to a lay person.*[24]

In England and Wales there is considerable interest in providing patients with the performance statistics of hospitals and clinicians. In the future such information may be used as part of the process whereby patients make an informed choice about their treatment. In 1996, the Florida legislature enacted the Patient's Right to Know Act.[25] This Act gives patients the additional right to know the following:

- the number of patients in each Diagnosis-Related Group (DRG) . . . for which the provider discharged at least 25 patients during the preceding calendar year
- the mortality rate for each DRG
- the infection rate for each DRG.[25]

Present situation in other jurisdictions

When 'informed consent' is seen as integral to good clinical care, it frequently becomes part of statute law. In Ontario, the Health Care Consent Act, 1996 recognised the need:

    1 (a) to provide rules with respect to treatment that apply
        consistently in all settings . . .
      (c) to enhance the autonomy of persons for whom treatment
        is proposed . . .
      (d) to promote communication and understanding between
        health practitioners and their patients or clients.[26]

However, in contrast to some states in the USA, as yet there has been no attempt to define which risks and side-effects are material, or to specify which ones must be disclosed.

    The most effective way of ensuring the rights of patients is to incorporate them into a separate law. By spelling out the legal rights of patients in a single legal instrument. they become readily accessible, transparent and enforceable. This has happened in the following countries:

- Finland – law on the legal status and rights of patients (1992)
- The Netherlands – Medical Assistance Act (1994)
- Lithuania – law on the rights of patients and damage done to patients (1996)
- Iceland – law on the rights of patients (1997)
- Denmark – law on the rights of patients (1998).[27]

The gradual spread of such laws across Europe, together with their acceptance in the USA and Canada, is likely to influence both Government policy and pressure groups that wish to improve patient care in England and Wales. The Medical Assistance Act in The Netherlands confirms all of the basic concepts of informed consent. In addition to providing information, healthcare professionals are required to listen to patients' needs and to take decisions together. The purpose is to create a friendly atmosphere in which patients will not be overwhelmed. Additional support comes from interpreters for patients for whom Dutch is not their first language.[28] The incorporation of such ideas into statute law is likely to have a profound effect on the delivery of care in countries such as The Netherlands. If introduced in England and Wales, it would formulate practice in Government hospitals, even with limited funding.

    In the same year as the Medical Assistance Act was enacted, the World Health Organization European Consultation on the Rights of Patients met in Amsterdam. Its purpose was to encourage co-operation between the European Union, the Council of Europe and the World Health Organization, and so to promote and protect the rights of patients. This was in response to work which showed that:

there are shared principles that are being adopted in a number of countries and which seem to be independent of the characteristics of a given country's health system.[29]

This is certainly true of informed consent. The meeting endorsed a document entitled *Principles of the Rights of Patients in Europe*. Although it has no legal standing, it does embody the aspirations of many European organisations about the future direction of healthcare and informed consent:

> *2.2 Patients have the right to be fully informed about their health status, including the medical facts about their condition, about the proposed medical procedures, together with the potential risks and benefits of each procedure; about alternatives to the proposed procedures, including the effect of non-treatment; and about diagnosis, prognosis and progress of treatment.*
>
> *2.3 Information may only be withheld from patients exceptionally when there is good reason to believe that this information would without any expectation of obvious positive effects cause them serious harm.*[29]

There is a general trend towards an acknowledgement that patients should know the details of procedures and treatments and the risks associated with them. Within Europe this can be seen in the Draft Charter of Fundamental Rights of the European Union. Article 3, section 2 states that:

> *In the fields of medicine and biology, the following must be respected in particular:*
> *– the free and informed consent of the person concerned, according to the procedures laid down by law.*[30]

Its success would depend on the law laying down adequate procedures. The evidence from several states in the USA would suggest that the creation of specific statutes to cover consent, and their support by statutory bodies which would define the type of disclosures that must be made, would resolve some of the lack of clarity that currently exists in England and Wales. It would ensure that clinicians knew what they must tell patients.

References

1 *Bolam v Friern Hospital Management Committee* [1957] 1 WLR 582–94.

2 *Bolitho v City & Hackney Health Authority* [1997] 4 All ER 771, HL (quoted in Stauch M, Wheat K and Tingle J (1998) *Sourcebook on Medical Law.* Cavendish Publishing Ltd, London).

3 *Salgo v Leland Stanford Junior University Board of Trustees* [1957] 317 P.2d 170, 181 (Cal. Dist. Ct. App. 1957).

4 *Re HIV Haemophiliac Litigation* [1990] NLJR 1349.

5 *Hill v Chief Constable of Yorkshire* [1989] AC 53.

6 Department of Health (2001) *Reference Guide to Consent for Examination or Treatment.* Department of Health, London.

7 Anon. (2001) NHS paternalism must go, says Milburn. *Daily Telegraph.* **30 January**: 8.

8 *Caroline Smith v National Health Service Litigation Authority* [2000] LTL 28/11/2000: [2001] Lloyd's Rep Med 90.

9 Harpwood V (2001) *Negligence in Healthcare. Clinical claims and risk.* Informa Publishing Group, London.

10 McLean S (1999) *Old Law, New Medicine. Medical ethics and human rights.* Rivers Oram Press, London.

11 Department of Health (1991) *The Patient's Charter.* Department of Health, London.

12 Department of Health (2001) *Consent. What you have a right to expect. A guide for adults;* http://www.doh.gov.uk/consent/adultconsent.htm. It includes the following advice:
> *How much do I need to know?*
> Some people want to know as much as possible about their condition and possible treatments; others prefer to leave decisions to the experts. No one providing healthcare will force information on you, for example, about the risks of treatment if you don't want to know. But remember, the person in the best position to know what matters most to you is *you* yourself.
> Perhaps you're the kind of person who is prepared to take some risks if there is also a chance of a very good outcome. On the other hand, you might rather put up with some discomfort than have treatment which carries a small risk of making things worse – even though it ought to improve your condition. Only you can know what is important to you.

13 Patient Concern (2001) *How to Survive Surgery;* www.patientconcern.org.uk.

14 *Patient Agreement to Investigation, Treatment or Operation,* http://www.doh.gov.uk.

15 NHS Litigation Authority (2000) *Clinical Risk Management Standards June 2000*. Clinical Negligence Scheme for Trusts, Bristol.

16 Department of Health (2001) *Seeking Consent: working with older people*. Department of Health, London.

17 General Medical Council (2001) *Good Medical Practice May 2001*. General Medical Council, London.

18 General Medical Council (1998) *Seeking Patients' Consent: the ethical considerations*. General Medical Council, London.

19 United Kingdom Central Council for Nursing, Midwifery and Health Visiting (1996) *Guidelines for Professional Practice*. United Kingdom Central Council for Nursing, Midwifery and Health Visiting, London.

20 British Society of Gastroenterology (1999) *Guidelines for Informed Consent for Endoscopic Procedures*. British Society of Gastroenterology, London.

21 BRI Inquiry (July 2001) *Final Report. The inquiry into the management of care of children receiving complex heart surgery at the Bristol Royal Infirmary*. Bristol Royal Infirmary Inquiry Command Paper CM 5207; http://www.bristol-inquiry.org.uk.

22 Louisiana Uniform Consent Law – La. R.S. 40: 1299.40 (http://www.legis.state.la.us/tsrs).

23 *Hondroulis v Schumacher* [1989] 553 So 2d 398 (La. 1989) (quoted in http://www.intrepidresources.com . . . informed_consent.htm p.2).

24 Medical Liability and Insurance Improvement Act of Texas, 1979, Art. 4590i. Vernon's Texas Civil Statutes.

25 The Patient's Right to Know Act of 1996, Florida.

26 Health Care Consent Act, 1996 S.O. 1996, c.2, Sched A.

27 Hungarian Civil Liberties Union (HCLU) Policy Papers. Policy paper on the rights of patients; http://www.c3.hu/~hclu/publ-3.htm.

28 Koster N (1997) *Patient Rights and Patient Education in The Netherlands*; http://www.nottingham.ac.uk/law/hrlc/hrnews/.../koster.ht.

29 *Principles of the Rights of Patients in Europe*; http://www.health.fgov.be/WH13/peri . . . /WWH19019804.ht.

30 Draft Charter of Fundamental Rights of the European Union: CHARTER 4470/1/00 REV 1 CONVENT 47.

Chapter 5

Consent to investigation: the role of information in consent processes

Introduction

During the past decade there has been significant growth in the number of information leaflets available for patients. This has been encouraged by the concepts of patient empowerment, the Patient's Charter, shorter hospital stays and greater health awareness. Consumerism and the emergence of self-help groups have also contributed. These developments are contrary to the medical tradition of Hippocrates, in which telling patients the truth about illness was not considered to be in their best interests.[1] In recent times, opposition to patient education has focused around the idea that such an approach will increase anxiety levels, raise consultation rates and prolong their duration. However, consent to procedures must be informed and risks must be acknowledged. Patients should be encouraged to get the most out of consultations by arriving with prepared lists of questions.[2]

Patient education services should enable both patients and their families to make informed decisions about their health, to manage their illness and to implement follow-up care at home. Interestingly, such an approach has been an essential component of nursing since the time of Florence Nightingale, and it is usually nurses who provide this service.

Written information is important because it provides a permanent record which is available for later consultation. However, if it is to be effective it must be noticed, read, understood, believed and remembered.[3] Surprisingly, until recently there has been little effort to ensure that patients understand what they receive, and there have been few attempts at evaluation.

The need of the patient to understand their disease so that they can effectively share in its management is critical to successful treatment in diabetes and asthma. When this need is absent, the drive to produce effective high-quality information and education programmes has been restricted to enthusiastic amateurs. However, as more and more medication becomes available over the counter, the associated commercialisation has ensured that new treatments are promoted directly to patients. Integral to this approach is the need to educate the general public about disease. Clinicians must be involved in the process if we are to ensure that information is accurate and interpretation is balanced.

Unfortunately, the sophistication of today's society is not always accompanied by an equivalent reading ability. Indeed, literary skills do not correlate with appearance, number of years of schooling or an individual's intelligence.[4,5] In practice there is often a significant educational gap between providers of health education and patients who consume it.[6-8] There is virtually no evidence about those factors which determine whether health-related information is noticed or read. In addition, patients frequently fail to understand their doctor because of cultural and ethnic differences.[6] Such differences can block any form of communication, yet in the worlds of marketing and education there has been considerable work on improved methods of teaching and information provision. Attractive material can be made available in the form of audio tapes and videos as well as booklets. However, the scientific evaluation of audio tapes and videos has been less rigorous, although media professionals monitor audiences to assess their response to commercial programmmes.[9] In the limited number of studies where evaluation has taken place, long-term knowledge gain has been very limited. However, there appears to be a good correlation between learning by listening and learning by reading. In this context, audio tapes can be particularly useful for the visually impaired, those for whom English is a second language and individuals with poor literary skills.[10] Videos would seem to have a specific place in skill building, where they can begin the process through demonstration.

As we move towards evidence-based treatment, critical evaluation of information and educational resources is needed, and the use of randomised controlled trials of their efficacy have just as much of a place here as in any other therapeutic approach.

Patient information

The success of educational packages for patients will depend on scientific evaluation and the demonstration that they influence the delivery and utilisation of care. Although some still believe that the purpose of patient education is greater compliance, Rankin and

Stallings[11] have highlighted the fact that education should allow patients to make informed choices, which can include non-compliance. They prefer the terms *adherence, concurrence* and *co-operation*, but this terminology is not yet widespread. Although it is unlikely that patient education will reduce mortality, there is evidence that adherence to treatment and increased awareness of side-effects will also have some benefit.[12] For example, Fordham[13] found that written information led to cleaner colons in those attending for barium enema X-rays. The meta-analysis of Mullen *et al.*[14] presented data on the effects of instructional and educational methods on adherence. Patients who were exposed to such interventions were significantly more adherent than those who had received no such education. Ideally, patients should be involved in all of the processes – from the identification of needs through to evaluation – and tests of readability, comprehension and recall should be included. Another outcome that can be evaluated is the ability of the patient to present him- or herself at the most propitious time for early diagnosis and treatment.[15] Before educational packages are marketed, they should be tested on representative patient samples and their effect on outcomes assessed by means of randomised controlled trials.

Production

A systematic approach should be adopted which is based on an evaluation of the needs of the patient[16] and the identification of those critical messages which clinicians wish to convey. Only in this way can effective and robust material be produced. In order to maximise the benefit for partially literate patients, the purpose of the material must be explained, its message should be logical, and it should relate to personal experience rather than make generalisations (*see* Tables 5.1 and 5.2).[17] The investigation by Michielutte *et al.*[18] of the role of illustrations showed significantly better comprehension by illiterate women of a pamphlet on cervical cancer when the text was complemented by relevant illustrations, although this has not always proved to be the case.[19–21] Moll *et al.*[22,23] studied the use of cartoons as aids to increasing knowledge, and recall of illustrated topics was found to be significantly poorer than recall of unillustrated ones. Unfortunately, the items accompanied by the cartoons were not varied experimentally, so these findings could reflect the fact that some of the information was more difficult to learn. Another possibility is that the illustrations distracted the readers. The role of illustrated material in patient education will inevitably change with the growth of videos and multi-media resources. The gap between the literate and illiterate may be narrowed, and it seems likely that discrepancies between various studies with regard to the use of illustrations will be resolved (*see* Tables 5.3 and 5.4).

Table 5.1: Essential criteria for good information

1 Has a well-defined target audience
2 Easily understood by the majority of recipients
3 Conveys clear messages
4 Produces a better understanding of disease processes
5 Improves the practices of the target audience
6 Reduces disease morbidity or even mortality
7 Increases patients' ability to cope with disease

Table 5.2: Effective writing for patients

- Write in a conversational style.
- Use short words and short sentences.
- Use direct questions.
- Be consistent with the use of words.
- Limit each paragraph to a single message.
- Use headers to alert readers to what is coming.
- Minimise information that is unrelated to the central concepts in the text.
- Use affirmative sentences most of the time.
- Use negative sentences to emphasise avoidance of an action.
- Place the most important information first or last.
- Ask patients to read your script and make suggestions.

Table 5.3: Stages in the development of patient information

Product formulation
Who is the audience?
What do they believe?
What is the purpose of the information?
How is the information best presented?

Product preparation
Develop prototypes.
Field-test prototypes.

Product verification
Pre-test target population with trial educational material.
If material achieves its aims, release for general use.

Product revision
Identify objectives that were not met during verification procedure.
Revise material.

Table 5.4: Good layout improves comprehension and readability

- Unjustified lines are easy to read.
- Indenting the first line of a paragraph increases the speed of reading.
- Type size should be at least 10 point.
- Capitals reduce the speed of comprehension.
- Italics reduce the speed of reading.
- Headings should be made to stand out by the use of different type faces or by inserting spaces.
- Use arabic numbers.

Evaluation

However, reading still remains the key to information for literate people, and at present those who cannot read operate on a more restricted information base.[24] The scientific evaluation of patient information must therefore include tests of both readability and comprehension.[25] However, the process should be a dynamic one which also investigates the long-term effects of the material.

Tests of readability

Readability encompasses the ease with which a piece of writing may be read. There are many formulae for assessing this (*see* Table 5.5).[26–32] They were originally designed as 'predictive averages' which could be used to rank the difficulty of books used in American schools. They are based on difficulties of vocabulary and average length of sentences, and they measure the character of a passage rather than the reader. In general, validation by this method has been used in the USA and on healthy people – the value and role of these formulae in other settings is less clear. The technical vocabulary of the health professions automatically creates problems, as many medical terms are polysyllabic.[33,34] In addition, readability formulae fail to take into account the interest and background of the reader (e.g. a patient with inflammatory bowel disease will know much of the vocabulary associated with that illness), so these formulae can overestimate the difficulty of a passage. Readability formulae also fail to take into account the reader's motivation and the meanings that may be derived from the context of well-written material.

Despite these reservations, readability measures are often used by health educators to ensure that their products can be understood by a wide cross-section of patients.[35] An adequate score is not a sufficient

Table 5.5: Common tests of readability of health-related literature

Readability test	Common use
Flesch Reading Ease[a]	Insurance industry
Flesch Kincaid Index[b]	USA Government and military
Dale–Chall formula[c,d]	
SMOG grading	USA health industry
(Simple Measure of Gobbledegook)[e]	
Gunning's FOG Index[f,g]	General reading assessment

These tests were developed using techniques such as McCall–Crabbs Standard Test Lessons in Reading Validation Exercise.
[a] Flesch RR (1948) A new readability yardstick. *J Appl Psychol.* **32**: 221–3.
[b] Flesch R (1974) *The Art of Readable Writing.* Harper & Row, New York.
[c] Dale E and Chall JS (1948) A formula for predicting readability. *Educ Res Bull.* **27**: 11–20.
[d] Dale E and Chall JS (1948) A formula for predicting readability: instructions. *Educ Res Bull.* **27**: 27–54.
[e] McLaughlin H (1969) Smog grading: a new readability formula. *J Reading.* **22**: 639–46.
[f] Gunning R (1968) The FOG index after twenty years. *J Bus Commun.* **6**: 3–13.
[g] Gunning R (1968) *The Technique of Clear Writing.* McGraw-Hill, New York.

indicator of good writing (e.g. good readability scores can be obtained by documents written in appalling style or with poorly chosen content). Bearing this proviso in mind, the use of *both* shorter words *and* shorter sentences is likely to increase comprehension, provided that the change in readability is large. If material is made too easy, it may become less acceptable to the more intelligent reader, although the evidence would not appear to support this view.[36]

Tests of comprehension

The Cloze technique[37–40] is a systematic test of comprehension. Every fifth word is omitted from a text while the first and last sentence are kept intact and proper nouns are retained throughout the piece under consideration. In total about 50 words are deleted from a text, and the candidate has to identify the exact word omitted rather than synonyms or equivalent phrases. The test assesses how much knowledge can be obtained from a text surrounding these blank spaces, and thus determines how well such information is used to obtain further information.[37]

$$\text{Comprehension score} = \frac{\text{raw score}}{\text{total number of blanks}} \times 100\%.$$

A score of 60% indicates that the piece was understood, while a score of

40–60% points to a need for some supplementary explanation in the text. A score of less than 40% shows that the passage was too difficult. The Cloze technique is probably the best method of assessing a document's value in patient education programmes, but has seldom been used in clinical studies. Possible reasons include the sense that this test is similar to an examination and that one can either pass or fail.

For some people, listening comprehension is better than reading comprehension, so it is more sensible for the text to be read out or an audio tape provided. However, there is no universally recognised technique for the subsequent measurement of listening comprehension.

Effectiveness of written information

About 70% of patients claim to have read information that was given to them. However, in 1964 Mohammed[41] showed that 33% of her sample of 220 patients drawn from a population of 300 diabetics were either unable to read or unable to comprehend printed health information written at the most basic level, and this finding has been confirmed repeatedly (*see* Table 5.6).[42] A further 10% were unable to see the information to read it, although this is likely to reflect diabetic eye disease rather than being true for the population in general. Such studies would suggest a need to make a formal check of a patient's reading ability prior to giving them printed information. Some of these patients will keep leaflets for future reference. Indeed, although patients forget much of the written information that is given to them, when it is understood it has the advantage of being available for future reference.

Table 5.6: Problems with written materials

- Not always noticed
- Not always read
- Not always understood
- Not always remembered

Effectiveness of video information

Rigorous scientific assessment of the educational value of patient videos is uncommon.[43,44] However, the extensive use of video technology in endoscopy and now in laparoscopy provides an opportunity for the production of instant personalised colour movies (*see* Table 5.7). In 1980, Parker[45] used such films to help patients to understand the procedures that they were about to undergo, and subsequently to show them precisely what had been done and why they should follow the discharge instructions even though they did not feel unwell. However, Levy *et al.*[46] were unable to show that such an approach reduced anxiety prior to the procedure.

Nowadays videos can be produced cheaply and tailor-made for a given patient population. In addition, they can ensure a standard level of teaching, and they are particularly useful when there is a high rate of functional illiteracy.

Table 5.7: Educational value of videos

- Present powerful role models of particular behaviour, attitudes and values.
- Present active illustrative material.
- Can be used to provide direct feedback of a learner patient's performance of complex tasks.

Measuring the long-term effects of patient education

The purpose of patient education is to change behaviour – for example, by promoting better adherence to treatment and increased co-operation with surveillance programmes. There are various methods by which learning can be measured:

1   direct observation of behaviour
2   rating scales and checklists
3   oral questioning
4   written assessment.

A further important aspect of assessment of the long-term consequences of educational material is the need to measure persistence of new knowledge.

Direct observation of behaviour

This is the most accurate method because it is well recognised that there is a clear difference between what people say they will do and what they actually do.[47] This technique is commonly used when assessing the acquisition of new skills (e.g. self-injection techniques).

Rating scales and checklists

Rating scales, which describe behaviour patterns in words, can be constructed to assess the effect of patient education programmes. The wording must be precise and the scale should include all pertinent points. One limiting factor is the number of levels of achievement that can be represented. A practical example which many doctors will have encountered is the Manchester Rating Scale, which is used to describe the behaviour of trainees in general practice.

A checklist is closely related to a rating scale. In such a list crucial steps in behaviour are chosen, and during its use each element of this behaviour is recorded as present or absent. Checklists also overcome some of the difficulties that are encountered in quantifying direct observation of behaviour. Both rating scales and checklists are best used for assessing activities (e.g. self-administration of injections) rather than understanding of disease and reasons for adherence to treatment.

Questionnaire tests of knowledge

Testing of patients' knowledge can be used to assess the effects of educational programmes. Tests may be constructed in a true/false format or use a multiple-choice format. They should present problems in a sequence from simple to complex and be appropriate for the patient's literary level. They need to be comprehensive and evaluate all of the major concepts involved in the subject under investigation. Their contents are best determined by consultation with nurses and physicians experienced in the field. This quality of a test is called *content validity*. The test score should also relate to actual patient behaviour in the present (*contemporary validity*) or the future (*predictive validity*) (i.e. does a test score correlate with good adherence to treatment and so better outcome?). If a test has a high degree of validity, its value for decision making will be greater.

One major problem with such tests is that they need to be updated as knowledge about a disease and its treatment increases. A good example of such an approach is the Kidney Disease Questionnaire which was devised by Devins *et al.*[48]

Conclusion

Patient education does not consist merely of needs assessment, information giving and its evaluation. It is an ongoing process which requires periodic reinforcement. Although physicians and the lay population may differ in their opinions about whether patients should be provided with emotionally charged information, various surveys have shown that the vast majority of people believe that they should be told if they have cancer or other fatal diseases. In practice, information can reduce anxiety levels and consultation rates.[49–51] Patients have a right to know about all aspects of their illness, and this knowledge must form the foundation for any therapeutic alliance between doctors, nurses and patients.

References

1 Bartlett EE (1986) Historical glimpses of patient education in the United States. *Patient Educ Counsel.* **8**: 135–49.

2 Meredith P, Emberton M and Wood C (1995) New direction in information for patients. More attention should be given to finding out what works. *BMJ.* **311**: 4–5.

3 Ley P (1992) *Communicating with Patients: improving communication, satisfaction and compliance.* Chapman and Hall, London.

4 Doak LG and Doak CC (1980) Patient comprehension profiles. Recent findings and strategies. *Patient Counsel Health Educ.* **2**: 101–6.

5 Schatzman L and Straass A (1955) Social class and moods of communication. *Am J Sociol.* **60**: 329–38.

6 Boyle CM (1970) Differences between patients and doctors. Interpretation of some common medical terms. *BMJ.* **2**: 286–9.

7 Anon. (1989) Write for your patient (editorial). *Lancet.* **1**: 1175.

8 Fletcher CM (1973) *Communication in Medicine.* Rock Carling Monograph. Nuffield Provincial Hospitals Trust, London.

9 Probert C, Frisby S and Mayberry JF (1991) The role of educational videos in gastroenterology. *J Clin Gastroenterol.* **13**: 620–21.

10 Meade CD, McKinney P and Barnas GP (1994) Educating patients with limited literary skills: the effectiveness of printed and videoed materials about colon cancer. *Am J Pub Health.* **84**: 119–21.

11 Rankin SH and Stallings KD (1990) *Patient Education: issues, principles and practices.* JB Lippincott, Philadelphia, PA.

12 Mazzuca SA (1982) Does patient education in chronic disease have therapeutic value? *J Chron Dis.* **35**: 521–9.

13 Fordham SD (1978) Increasing patient compliance in preparing for the barium enema examination. *Am J Radiol.* **133**: 913–15.

14 Mullen PD, Green LW and Persinger GS (1985) Clinical trials of patient education for chronic conditions. A comparative meta-analysis of intervention types. *Prev Med.* **14**: 753–81.

15 Redman BK (1992) *The Process of Patient Education.* Mosby Year Book, St Louis, MO.

16 Rees JEP, Mayberry JF and Calcraft B (1983) What the patient wants to know about Crohn's disease. *J Clin Gastroenterol.* **5**: 221–2.

17 Kanouse DE and Hayes-Roth B (1980) Cognitive considerations in the design of produce warnings. In: LA Morris, M Mazzis and I Barofsky (eds) *Banbury Report 6: product labelling and health risks.* Cold Spring Harbor Laboratories, Cold Spring Harbor, New York.

18 Michielutte R, Bahnson J, Dignan MB and Schroeder EM (1992) The use of illustrations and narrative text style to improve readability of a health education brochure. *J Cancer Educ.* **7**: 251–60.

19 Midgeley JM and Macrae AW (1971) Audiovisual media in general practice. *J R Coll Gen Pract.* **21**: 346–51.

20 Snowman J and Cunningham DJ (1975) A comparison of pictorial and written adjunct aids. *J Educ Psychol.* **67**: 307–11.

21 Willows DM (1978) A picture is not always worth a thousand words. *J Educ Psychol.* **70**: 255–62.

22 Moll JMH and Wright V (1972) Evaluation of the Arthritis and Rheumatism Council handbook on gout. *Ann Rheum Dis.* **31**: 405–11.

23 Moll JMH, Wright V, Jeffrey MR, Goode JD and Humberstone PM (1977) The cartoon in doctor–patient communication. *Ann Rheum Dis.* **36**: 225–31.

24 Doak CC, Doak LG, Root J et al. (1985) *Teaching Patients with Low Literacy Skills.* JB Lippincott Company, Philadelphia, PA.

25 Ley P, Goldman M, Bradshaw PW, Kincey JA and Walker C (1972) The comprehensibility of some X-ray leaflets. *J Inst Health Educ.* **10**: 47–53.

26 Flesch RR (1948) A new readability yardstick. *J Appl Psychol.* **32**: 221–3.

27 Flesch R (1974) *The Art of Readable Writing.* Harper & Row, New York.

28 Dale E and Chall JS (1948) A formula for predicting readability. *Educ Res Bull.* **27**: 11–20.

29 Dale E and Chall JS (1948) A formula for predicting readability: instructions. *Educ Res Bull.* **27**: 27–54.

30 McLaughlin H (1969) Smog grading: a new readability formula. *J Reading.* **22**: 639–46.

31 Gunning R (1968) The FOG index after twenty years. *J Bus Commun.* **6**: 3–13.

32 Gunning R (1968) *The Technique of Clear Writing*. McGraw-Hill, New York.

33 Pichert JW and Elam P (1985) Readability formulas may mislead you. *Patient Educ Counsel.* **7**: 181–91.

34 Wagenaar WA, Schreuder R and Wijlhuizen GJ (1987) Readability of instructional text written for the general public. *Appl Cogn Psychol.* **1**: 155–68.

35 Baker GC (1991) Writing easily read patient education handouts: a computerised approach. *Semin Dermatol.* **10**: 102–6.

36 Klare GR (1976) A second look at the validity of readability formulas. *J Read Behav.* **8**: 129–52.

37 Bormuth JR (1975) The cloze procedure: literacy in the classroom. In: *Help for the Reading Teacher: new directory for research*. National Conference in Research in English. National Institute of Education (DHEW), Washington DC, March 1975.

38 Holcomb CA (1983) The cloze procedure and readability of patient-oriented drug information. *J Drug Educ.* **13**: 347–57.

39 McKenna MC and Robinson RD (1980) *An Introduction to the Cloze Procedure. An annotated bibliography*. International Reading Association, Newark, DE.

40 Taylor WS (1953) Cloze procedure: a new test for measuring readability. *Journalism Q.* **30**: 415–33.

41 Mohammed M (1964) Patients' understanding of written health information. *Nurs Res.* **13**: 100–8.

42 Estey A, Musseau A and Keehn L (1991) Patient comprehension of printed health information. *Patient Educ Counsel.* **18**: 165–9.

43 Gagliano ME (1988) A literature review of the efficacy of videos in patient education. *J Med Educ.* **63**: 785–92.

44 Nielsen E and Sheppard MA (1988) Television as a patient education tool: a review of its effectiveness. *Patient Educ Counsel.* **11**: 3–16.

45 Parker CF (1981) Endoscopic movies for patient teaching. *AORN J.* **34**: 254–7.

46 Levy N, Landmann L, Stermer E, Erdreich M, Beny A and Meisels R (1989) Does a detailed explanation prior to gastroscopy reduce the patient's anxiety? *Endoscopy.* **21**: 263–5.

47 Hynam KA, Hart AR, Gay SR, Inglis A, Wicks ACB and Mayberry JF (1995) Screening for colorectal cancer: reasons for refusal of faecal occult blood testing in a general practice in England. *J Epidemiol Commun Health.* **49**: 84–6.

48 Devins GM, Binik YM, Mandin H *et al.* (1990) The Kidney Disease

Questionnaire: a test for measuring patient knowledge about end-stage renal disease. *J Clin Epidemiol.* **43**: 297–307.

49 Mayberry JF and Fisher N (1989) Use of patient information booklet on inflammatory bowel disease by family practitioners. *Ital J Gastroenterol.* **21**: 53–4.

50 Mayberry JF, Morris JS, Calcraft B and Rhodes J (1985) Information assessment by patients of a booklet on Crohn's disease. *Pub Health Lond.* **99**: 239–42.

51 Smart H, Mayberry JF, Calcraft B, Morris JS and Rhodes J (1986) Effect of information booklet in patients awaiting levels and consultation rates in Crohn's disease. *Pub Health Lond.* **100**: 184–6.

Chapter 6

Consent to investigation: an empirical study of information and consent processes in gastroscopy

Introduction

Consent to procedures is a practical problem that is faced every day by clinicians, for whom there are significant questions as to how much they should disclose about risk, especially because the courts have chosen not to specify a percentage. For one person a 1 in 1000 risk may be of no consequence, whereas for another it would stop them undergoing an intervention. Particular risks may be important for one person but not for another. One purpose of the study described in this chapter was to identify the level of risk which an average person would want to know for a simple diagnostic procedure. Here it is important to make a comparison with clinical negligence specialists, who advise patients, but who may view the requirements of consent in a way that is not consistent with its legal requirements. Clinicians would benefit from a knowledge of the risk that such specialists might consider to be significant. This knowledge could inform daily practice when discussing procedures with patients. At present no such information is available and doctors must rely on their clinical judgement. In addition to what patients should be told, there is limited information on when consent should be sought. The concept of a 'cooling off' period is popular in insurance contracts, and perhaps it should be considered in clinical settings as well.

In *Re C*,[1] one of the criteria required to establish that patients had the capacity to understand was that they could comprehend information. Professional bodies and other groups committed to the concept of informed consent recognise that information must be simple and presented in a form that patients can understand. In the study described here, the value of a standard information sheet written in easy-to-understand English was tested through simple 'Yes/No' questions. The ethical standards underlying consent, especially patient autonomy, require patients to understand what is to happen. If patients cannot understand information then doctors will have failed to reach the professional standards for consent required by bodies such as the General Medical Council. It could also be argued that the first of the three criteria needed in *Re C*[1] would not have been met.

Many of the cases concerned with inadequate consent occurred some time after the intervention. In addition to an initial misunderstanding of explanations about an intervention, the recall of patients (as well as that of clinicians) may be suspect. The use of a standard test in this study allowed the decline in memory of information about the intervention to be measured formally. The view that interventions are of major concern to patients, so they will vividly recall details, may not be correct.

This study also allowed an investigation of linguistic difficulties which may limit the validity of consent. It was conducted among South Asian patients with a working knowledge of English, rather than among individuals who were unable to speak the language. If differences exist between English and South Asian responses, the need for adequate translation is apparent.

If patients 'fail' the test of comprehension, for whatever reason, can they give consent to the procedure? This is not a question of whether they have capacity, but rather of whether, having capacity, they have been properly informed. If they have not been informed, can they give consent? If they lack even the broadest understanding of the procedure, could clinicians be guilty of battery?

Method

Requirements for informed consent

A total of 100 consecutive patients who had undergone gastroscopy in the previous two months were asked to complete a postal questionnaire about aspects of the consent procedure. The questionnaire dealt with the following:

- what they ought to have been told about the test
- when patients ought to be told
- how they ought to have been told
- how often they ought to be told

- the level of risk that ought to be discussed
- the need or otherwise to sign a consent form
- the need or otherwise to check on patients' understanding of the test.

An identical questionnaire was also sent to senior partners in 149 solicitor practices throughout England and Wales who held a clinical negligence franchise from the Legal Aid Board in 2000.

Further information about endoscopists

In addition, 100 consecutive patients who were about to undergo a gastroscopy were asked to complete a questionnaire concerning the details that they wanted about their endoscopist. This questionnaire dealt with the following:

- level of expertise – whether trained or in training and supervised
- length of expertise – number of years trained and number of endoscopies performed each year
- complaints against endoscopist
- type of endoscopist – nurse or doctor.

The information leaflets

An information leaflet was prepared for patients who were about to undergo a diagnostic gastroscopy. The first version dealt with the following four issues.

- Why do I need this test?
- How is the test done?
- How long will the test take?
- How safe is the test?

The leaflet was written in easy-to-read English. Its length was 302 words, and 87% of the words were two syllables or less in length. The average length of sentences was 8.2 words. The Flesch Reading Ease score was 75.3, which puts it in the 'fairly easy' category.[2] The FOG Index was 7.6, which means that the level of difficult words present in the text should have made it understandable to an 11-year-old.[3]

Patients were asked to identify whether four statements were 'True' or 'False'. These questions were based on the content of the leaflet. The statements were as follows.

- The endoscope can be used to find the cause of indigestion.
- The test is usually done under a general anaesthetic.

- The test usually takes less than ten minutes.
- The test is perfectly safe and never has any risks.

The answers to these questions were present in the text. In the first version the word 'indigestion' was not used, although 'stomach pains' were referred to. After an initial group of patients had been studied, a second version of the leaflet was prepared. In this version the word 'indigestion' was included at the beginning of a list of reasons why gastroscopy may be performed. In this later version the text read as follows: 'It is used to find the cause of indigestion, stomach pains, weight loss and bleeding'.

Scoring of test statements

Of the four statements, two were correct or 'True' and two were incorrect or 'False'. A score of +1 was given for a correct answer and a score of −1 for an incorrect answer. No response was scored as 0. For each leaflet a patient could score between −4 (all answers wrong) and +4 (all answers right). In addition to this more comprehensive measure of understanding, where negative marking was used, a second score was recorded which took the form of a simple addition of all of the correct answers.

Population studied

The leaflets were given to consecutive patients who attended the Endoscopy Unit at Leicester General Hospital for a diagnostic gastroscopy. Each patient was given the leaflet to read prior to the examination and asked to answer the four questions unaided. Details of the patient's age and ethnic background (European or South Asian) were recorded at the time of completion of the questionnaire. If a patient answered the questions incorrectly, the right answers were explained to the patient before seeking their written consent and proceeding with the endoscopy.

Six months after the patients had completed the questions attached to the second version of the leaflet, about half of them were sent an identical group of questions by post. In addition, this group of patients was asked whether they could recall seeing the leaflet at the time of their endoscopy, if it had been helpful, and when they felt it would be best given to patients.

Table 6.1: Responses from patients and from solicitors specialising in clinical negligence to a questionnaire about information and informed consent

Question	Patients (n = 81)	Solicitors (n =79)	x^2	Degrees of freedom	Significance
When is it best to tell the patient details of the test?					
Two weeks before	36	59			
The day before	17	11	21.7	3	< 0.0001
An hour before	8	4.5			
Immediately before	18	1.5			
How often should patients be told about the test?					
Just once	56	10			
On two different occasions	23	62	53.5	2	< 0.0001
On three different occasions	1	6			
How should patients be told about the test?					
By a nurse	34	25			
By a doctor	31	39			
By the doctor who does the test	58	50	22.2	4	< 0.0002
By means of a booklet	29	62			
By means of a video	7	28			

Patients who had undergone gastroscopy and solicitors who were specialists in clinical negligence were asked to complete identical questionnaires about aspects of the provision of information and timing of the consent procedure. The difference between solicitors and patients with regard to the methods of providing information is due to the solicitors' choice of a booklet ($x^2 = 27.9$, $P < 0.0001$) or a video ($x^2 = 15.3$, $P < 0.0001$).
Numbers do not always add up to n because not all respondents answered every question, and in the case of the question about how the patients should be told, they were asked to tick as many categories as they felt were useful.

Results

In total, 81 out of 100 patients (81% response rate) completed the questionnaire about the provision of information and obtaining informed consent. A similar questionnaire was returned by 79 of the 149 senior partners in solicitor practices which held a clinical negligence franchise (53% response rate) (*see* Table 6.1). A total of 75% of the solicitors felt that consent should be obtained two weeks before the procedure, compared with 44% of patients. This difference was statistically significant ($x^2 = 21.7$, $P < 0.0001$) and could be linked with the solicitors' view that patients should be told about the test on at least two occasions (86% compared with 30% of patients). Most patients (72%) wanted to receive information from the doctor who performed the test, whereas the solicitors slightly favoured a booklet (79%). Videos were also significantly more popular with solicitors than with patients as a means of providing information (*see* Table 6.1).

Clinical negligence solicitors and patients had different views about the type of information that patients should receive as part of the informed consent procedure. Solicitors believed that:

- patients should know why the test is needed (100% of respondents)
- patients should know the common dangers of the test (98.7% of respondents)
- patients should know how the test is performed (97.5% of respondents).

These values were all significantly higher than for the patient group. However, similar numbers of specialist solicitors (48%) and patients (38%) thought that patients should be told about very uncommon risks and dangers of gastroscopy (*see* Table 6.2).

Table 6.2: Responses by patients and by solicitors specialising in clinical negligence to questions about the type of information needed as part of the informed consent procedure

Question	Patients (n = 81)	Solicitors (n = 79)	χ^2	Significance
Why is the test needed?	73	79	6.2	<0.01
How is the test done?	53	77	24.9	<0.0001
What are the common dangers of the test?	59	78	19.7	<0.0001
What are the very uncommon risks and dangers of the test?	31	38	1.2	NS

Patients who had undergone a gastroscopy and solicitors who were specialists in clinical negligence were asked to complete an identical questionnaire on aspects of the provision of information and the timing of the consent procedure.
Numbers do not always add up to *n* because not all respondents answered every question.
NS, statistically non-significant.

The level of risk that should be routinely discussed is shown in Table 6.3. In total, 83% of patients wished to know about risks greater than 1 in 1000, whereas 58% of specialist solicitors believed that patients should be made aware of risks of less than 1 in 10 000. Indeed, 16% of specialist solicitors believed that patients should be made aware of risks of 1 in 1 million, compared with 6% of the patient group (*see* Table 6.3).

Both patients and clinical negligence solicitors strongly believed that patients should sign consent forms before undergoing procedures such as a gastroscopy. Both groups believed that there should be some method of formally checking whether patients understand what they have been told in the consent process (*see* Table 6.4).

Of the 100 patients who were asked to give details of the extra information that they would like to receive about their endoscopist, all

Table 6.3: Level of risk identified by patients and by solicitors specialising in clinical negligence as being appropriate to informed consent for a gastroscopy

Level of risk	Patients (n = 81) (%)	Solicitors (n = 79) (%)
1 in 10	53	4
1 in 100	15	16
1 in 1000	15	22
1 in 10 000	4	27
1 in 100 000	5	15
1 in 1 000 000	6	16

Patients and solicitors were asked to identify the frequency of serious complications which should be routinely disclosed to patients.

Table 6.4: Patients' and solicitors' views on signing consent forms and checking patients' understanding of the procedure

Question	Patients (n = 81)	Solicitors (n = 79)	χ^2	P-value
Should consent forms be signed?	72	78	5	< 0.02
Should patients' understanding be checked?	79	75	0.2	NS

Patients and solicitors completed a questionnaire about the signing of consent forms and the formal checking of patients' understanding of procedures. Seven patients had no views on signing consent forms, and two did not express an opinion on the formal checking of patients' understanding of procedures.
NS, statistically non-significant.

replied. In total, 69% wanted to know whether the practitioner was fully trained and 39% wanted to know the annual number of complaints registered against him or her. However, the majority of patients wanted the procedure performed immediately, rather than delaying in order to have it done by a trained practitioner or by a doctor in preference to a nurse.

A total of 168 patients received the first version of the gastroscopy leaflet, of whom 39 patients were of South Asian origin and were an average of 12 years younger than the English patients. The South Asian patients were able to read the leaflet, but had significantly lower scores in response to the four questions related to the gastroscopy procedure (see Table 6.5). The mean correct score with negative marking is probably a better indicator of overall understanding, and for English

Table 6.5: Responses to the first edition of an information leaflet on gastroscopies by English and Asian patients (n = 168)

	English patients	Asian patients	Student's t-test	z	P-value
Total (n)	129	39			
Age (years)	59	47	4.2		<0.0001
Mean total number of correct answers	3.2	2.7	3.6		<0.0004
Mean number of correct answers with negative marking for wrong answers	2.6	1.5	4		<0.0001
Questions answered correctly					
1 The endoscope can be used to find the cause of indigestion	78	24		−0.12	NS
2 The test is usually done under a general anaesthetic	122	23		5.7	<0.0001
3 The test usually takes less than ten minutes	107	30		0.85	NS
4 The test is perfectly safe and never has any risks	111	25		3.06	<0.002

A total of 168 patients were given an information leaflet about gastroscopies and then asked to answer four questions with a 'True/False' answer. The questions were at the end of the leaflet, and all answers were given in the text.
NS, statistically non-significant.

patients was 2.6 (range −4 to +4), compared with 1.5 (range −4 to +4) for South Asian patients. In the revised version the question about the safety of the test continued to be poorly answered, with 12% of patients failing to identify that this statement was false.

How effectively was this information retained over a period of six months? In total, 33 out of 43 patients who were sent the same four questions about the revised gastroscopy leaflet replied. The answers after six months were compared using a matched-pairs technique, and in addition the initial answers of the non-responders were compared with the initial answers of the responders. The responders and non-responders had comparable scores at the beginning of the study. After six months, the patients who had received the revised gastroscopy leaflet scored significantly lower than immediately after reading the leaflet. The mean correct score with negative marking fell from 3.6 to 2.7 (Mann–Whitney U-test $= 2.7$, $P < 0.007$).

Discussion

This study shows that most patients wanted to receive information about a test from the doctor who would be performing it, and that this should happen two weeks before the test. Significant numbers of patients wanted to know why the test was needed and the common dangers associated with it. In total, 83% of patients wanted risks of 1 in 1000 or higher to be disclosed. More than 50% of the patients also wanted to know whether the endoscopist was trained or a trainee. In comparison, 78% of solicitors believed that the test should be discussed with patients on at least two occasions and supported by booklets. Moreover, in sharp contrast, 31% of solicitors believed that serious risks of less than 1 in 100 000 should be disclosed routinely, compared with only 11% of patients. In *Sidaway v Board of Governors of the Bethlehem Royal Hospital & Maudsley Hospital & Others*,[4] Lord Diplock discussed the volunteering of unsought information by doctors and wrote:

> To decide what risks the existence of which a patient should be voluntarily warned . . . is as much an exercise of profes-sional skill and judgement as any other part of the doctor's comprehensive duty of care to the individual patient.[4]

The House of Lords had placed the responsibility for discussing risks on doctors. Lord Woolf said that significant risk could not be expressed in percentages, and recognised that flexibility was needed. In contrast, in Canada *Reibl v Hughes*[5] recognised that a 10% risk of a grave adverse event should be discussed voluntarily with patients. In total, 53% of patients in this study would agree with that figure. In contrast, in the Australian case of *Rogers v Whitaker*[6] when specific questions were asked by the patient, failure to discuss a risk of 1 in 14 000 was found to be negligent. In England and Wales, solicitors may consider failure to warn of very rare events as a possible case for litigation. If a subjective test for disclosure was adopted in England and Wales, as it has been in Australia, the view of solicitors who believe in disclosure of a risk of 1 in 1 million could significantly influence patients. The solution in some states in the USA has been to define which rare events should be disclosed, and thus to remove some of the uncertainty with which clinicians have to practise daily, both in the UK and in Australia.

In total, 98% of patients and 95% of solicitors believe that there ought to be formal testing of patients' understanding of information that is provided as part of the consent process. Such views fit well with an autonomous view of consent, and especially with the transatlantic doctrine of informed consent. In *Pearce v United Bristol Healthcare NHS Trust*[7] and *Gillian Carver v Hammersmith & Queen Charlotte's Special Health Authority*,[8] the importance of the intelligibility of information was central to the case. Kennedy and Grubb recognised that competence to give consent depended on the capacity to understand, rather than on actual understanding.[9] However, this in turn depended on the provision of adequate information. This study shows that even simple documents can fail to provide clear messages for patients, and that understanding can be radically affected by relatively small changes in the text. However, the use of such documents does provide clinicians with an opportunity to identify areas where knowledge is defective and to correct these. Such an approach is very much in line with Government policy, as well as with professional organisations such as the General Medical Council and the UKCC. The General Medical Council document, *Seeking Patients' Consent: the ethical considerations*,[10] views consent as a process. The use of a 'test' allows checks on understanding, opportunities for feedback and discussion, and documentation within the clinical record of the patient's understanding of any intervention. This record can be useful if there is later dispute about the information given, as memory does fade, as has been shown in this and other studies.[11–16] This finding might support the argument that patients later forget what they had once understood, particularly when it is assumed that most people will have the capability to give consent. In addition, solicitors' support for signed consent forms and tests of comprehension might suggest that they believe their absence could indicate a failure to discuss interventions and obtain consent.

Cultural background can also affect understanding.[17] Asians performed less well than English patients, with lower overall scores. In a study of patients in Delhi, 68% were able to recall details that they had been given prior to surgery, but the old, the poor and the less well educated performed significantly less well.[18] In the Medical Liability and Insurance Improvement Act of Texas,[19] the needs of Spanish speakers who were about to undergo hysterectomy were recognised, as was the need for translators in the Dutch Medical Assistance Act.[20] Such needs have now been recognised in the new consent form for use in England and Wales. It is arguable from cases outside the medical arena that without this support consent may be invalid.[21–23]

Consent has two functions in the doctor–patient relationship. One role is legal, in that it prevents charges of battery and trespass to the person being laid against the doctor or nurse. The other role is a clinical one, which secures patients' trust and co-operation.[24] In order to achieve a good ethical standard, the consent process should include details of the procedure, its purpose, complications, risks and alternatives. This study shows that, on a practical level, consent forms should be piloted on patients to ensure adequate levels of readability and understanding. If patients are to weigh information in the balance, they need to comprehend that information, and a formal test of its comprehension would allow doctors to correct misunderstandings. Their inclusion within the clinical record will limit clinicians' liability and help to demonstrate that discussions with a patient had taken place. From an ethical standpoint, consent needs to become an active process in which patients make *informed decisions* based on adequate information which is properly understood.

References

1 *Re C (adult refusal of treatment)* [1994] 1 WLR 290.
2 Flesch R (1949) *The Art of Readable Writing.* Harper and Brothers Publishers, New York.
3 Gunning R (1952) *The Technique of Clear Writing.* McGraw Hill, New York.
4 *Sidaway v Bethlehem Royal Hospital Governors* [1985] AC 871.
5 *Reibl v Hughes* [1980] 2 SCR 880, 114 DLR 93d, 1 14 CCLT 1, Can SC.
6 *Rogers v Whitaker* [1992] 175 CLR 479, 109 ALR 625, 16 BMLR 148.
7 *Pearce v United Bristol Healthcare NHS Trust* [1999] 48 BMLR 118.
8 *Gillian Karen Carver v Hammersmith & Queen Charlotte's Special Health*

Authority [2000] QBD (Nelson J0 25/2/2000) LTL 10/4/2000 (unreported elsewhere).

9 Kennedy I and Grubb A (1994) *Medical Law* (2e). Butterworths, London.

10 General Medical Council (1998) *Seeking Patients' Consent: the ethical considerations*. General Medical Council, London.

11 Cassileth BR, Zupkis RV, Sutton-Smith K and March V (1980) Informed consent – why are its goals imperfectly realized? *NEJM.* **302**: 896–900.

12 Lavelle-Jones C, Byrne DJ, Rice P and Cuschieri A (1993) Factors affecting quality of informed consent. *BMJ.* **306**: 885–90.

13 Proctor DD, Price J, Mihas BS, Gumber SC and Christie EM (1999) Patient recall and appropriate timing for obtaining informed consent for endoscopic procedures. *Am J Gastroenterol.* **94**: 967–71.

14 Elfant AB, Korn C, Mendez L, Pello MJ and Peikin SR (1995) Recall of informed consent after endoscopic procedures. *Dis Colon Rectum.* **38**: 1–3.

15 Agre P (1993) *A Trial of Methods of Instructing Patients to Meet Informed Consent Guidelines for Colonoscopy* (patient education videotape). EdD, Columbia University Teachers' College, New York.

16 Agre P, McKeee K, Gargon N and Kurtz RC (1997) Patient satisfaction with an informed consent process. *Cancer Pract.* **5**: 162–7.

17 Saw KC, Wood AM, Murphy K, Parry JR and Hartfall WG (1994) Informed consent: an evaluation of patients' understanding and opinion (with respect to the operation of transurethral resection of the prostate). *J R Soc Med.* **87**: 143–4.

18 Sanwal AK, Kumar S, Sahni P and Nundy S (1996) Informed consent in Indian patients. *J R Soc Med.* **89**: 196–8.

19 Medical Liability and Insurance Improvement Act of Texas, 1979, Art. 4590i. Vernon's Texas Civil Statutes.

20 Koster N (1997) *Patient Rights and Patient Education in the Netherlands*; http://www.nottingham.ac.uk/law/hrlc/hrnews/ . . . /koster.ht.

21 *Kunnath v The State* [1993] 4 All ER 30: [1993] 1 WLR 1315: [1993] 98 CAR 455: Guardian 20/8/93: [1993] 137 SJ(LB) 195: (1993) 143 NLJ 1332: TLR 30/7/93.

22 *Lloyds Bank plc v Waterhouse* [1990] ILR 27/2/90: [1991] 10 Tr LR: [1992] 2 FLR 97: [1991] 2 Fam Law 23.

23 *Hamid Dedsahti Haghighat* [1999] LTL 27/10/99 Extempore (unreported elsewhere).

24 *Re W* [1992] 4 All ER 627, 633.

Chapter 7

Conclusions and recommendations

Consent allows clinicians to conduct everyday clinical practice. It means that invasive procedures can be carried out without fear of allegations of assault or trespass. It establishes a relationship of mutual trust in which the patient believes that the clinician will work in his or her best interest and the clinician believes that the patient will accept his or her good faith. During the past century the balance in this relationship shifted from the paternalistic physician towards the autonomous patient. This change has required a more open relationship, with patients needing to know the true prognosis of their disease and the risks associated with any investigation or treatment.

Consent requires patients to have capacity, and this has been defined in *Re C*[1] as having the following three elements:

* comprehension and retention of information
* believing the information
* ability to weigh the information in the balance and make a choice.

If these three elements are present, the patient is able to agree to procedures, and for most people this will be the case. It is the practitioner's responsibility to ensure that the patient does have capacity.

Although the law requires doctors and nurses to give sufficient information to allow patients to make a decision about proposed interventions, within the UK 'informed consent' is not a legal requirement. However, case law is evolving. It will be influenced by human rights legislation and indirectly by the standards set by professional groups. Indeed, the Department of Health, professional bodies and specialist societies have increasingly accepted this transatlantic doctrine as the standard for reasonable practice. This movement towards informed consent by the professions may ultimately lead English courts to accept such consent as standard on the principles identified in Bolam and Bolitho.

The tension that currently exists between informed consent and legal practice means that clinicians are often uncertain about what level of risk to discuss with patients, and about the difference between general risks and those of specific concern to an individual patient. In *Sidaway*[2] it was decided that the amount of information that was given to a patient was not a matter of meeting objective criteria, but for the doctor to decide in individual cases. In *Pearce v United Bristol Healthcare NHS Trust* [1999],[3] the Court was concerned to say it was not possible to express 'significant risk' in percentage terms. This approach contrasts with many other jurisdictions, where the nature of information about risks and complications is defined by a statutory body which regularly reviews clinical procedures. In some jurisdictions, such as the USA, consent has been simplified for clinicians when specialist state boards have identified specific complications. In contrast, in England and Wales the decision as to what level of risk should be discussed has been left within professional discretion by the courts. Each case will be judged on its individual merits. In this uncertain situation, doctors and nurses need clear guidelines on consent, and those produced by the Department of Health[4] have leaned heavily in favour of 'informed consent'.

The analysis of case law and the empirical study reported in this book would suggest that the essential elements of consent that are needed include the following:

- discussions of the intervention at an early stage, some time prior to its delivery
- a simple explanation of the procedure – this should include its purpose, recognised complications and risks, as well as alternatives
- checks with the patient with regard to how much they wish to know, including what level and type of risk might concern them
- rechecking the patient's agreement to the intervention at a later stage, prior to the procedure
- frequent checking at all stages that the patient has understood what has been said
- documentation of these discussions throughout the clinical record.

Although informed consent has not yet been adopted in England and Wales, there has been a general move within healthcare in the UK towards greater patient involvement. This means that decisions made by the patient will need to be based on better information, and that rather than informed consent there will be informed decisions made by an autonomous patient.

References

1   *Re C (adult refusal of treatment)* [1994] 1 WLR 290.
2   *Sidaway v Bethlehem Royal Hospital Governors* [1984] 1 QB 493, 1 All ER 1018, CA.
3   *Pearce v United Bristol Healthcare NHS Trust* [1999] 48 BMLR 118.
4   Department of Health (2001) *Reference Guide to Consent for Examination or Treatment*. Department of Health, London.

Further reading and resources

Books and articles

- Agre P (1993) *A Trial of Methods of Instructing Patients to Meet Informed Consent Guidelines for Colonoscopy* (patient education videotape). EdD, Columbia University Teachers' College, New York.
- Agre P, McKeee K, Gargon N and Kurtz RC (1997) Patient satisfaction with an informed consent process. *Cancer Pract.* **5**: 162–7.
- Anon. (1989) Write for your patient (editorial). *Lancet.* **1**: 1175.
- Anon. (2001) NHS paternalism must go, says Milburn. *Daily Telegraph.* **30 January**: 8.
- Appelbaum PS, Lidz CW and Meisel A (1987) *Informed Consent. Legal theory and clinical practice.* Oxford University Press, New York.
- Baker GC (1991) Writing easily read patient education handouts: a computerised approach. *Semin Dermatol.* **10**: 102–6.
- Bartlett EE (1986) Historical glimpses of patient education in the United States. *Patient Educ Counsel.* **8**: 135–49.
- Beauchamp TL and Childress JF (2001) *Principles of Biomedical Ethics* (5e). Oxford University Press, Oxford.
- Bennett P (1999) Understanding responses to risk: some basic findings. In: P Bennett and K Calman (eds) *Risk Communication and Public Health.* Oxford University Press, Oxford.
- Bormuth JR (1975) The cloze procedure: literacy in the classroom. In: *Help for the Reading Teacher: new directory for research.* National Conference in Research in English. National Institute of Education (DHEW), Washington DC, March 1975.
- Boyle CM (1970) Differences between patients and doctors. Interpretation of some common medical terms. *BMJ.* **2**: 286–9.
- Bristol Royal Infirmary Secretariat (1999) *BRI Inquiry Paper on Informed Consent: concept, guidelines and practice with reference to children undergoing complex heart surgery.* BRI Secretariat, Bristol.
- British Society of Gastroenterology (1999) *Guidelines for Informed Consent for Endoscopic Procedures.* British Society of Gastroenterology, London.

- Brooke H and Barton A (2000) Consent to treatment. In: M Powers and N Harris (eds) *Clinical Negligence*. Butterworths, London.
- Calman KC and Royston GHD (1997) Risk language and dialects. *BMJ*. **315**: 939–42.
- Cassileth BR, Zupkis RV, Sutton-Smith K and March V (1980) Informed consent – why are its goals imperfectly realized? *NEJM*. **302**: 896–900.
- Dale E and Chall JS (1948) A formula for predicting readability. *Educ Res Bull*. **27**: 11–20.
- Dale E and Chall JS (1948) A formula for predicting readability: instructions. *Educ Res Bull*. **27**: 27–54.
- Department of Health (1991) *The Patient's Charter*. Department of Health, London.
- Department of Health (2001) *Reference Guide to Consent for Examination or Treatment*. Department of Health, London.
- Department of Health (2001) *Seeking Consent: working with older people*. Department of Health, London.
- Devins GM, Binik YM, Mandin H *et al.* (1990) The Kidney Disease Questionnaire: a test for measuring patient knowledge about end-stage renal disease. *J Clin Epidemiol*. **43**: 297–307.
- Doak CC, Doak LG, Root J *et al.* (1985) *Teaching Patients with Low Literacy Skills*. JB Lippincott Company, Philadelphia, PA.
- Doak LG and Doak CC (1980) Patient comprehension profiles. Recent findings and strategies. *Patient Counsel Health Educ*. **2**: 101–6.
- Draft Charter of Fundamental Rights of the European Union: CHARTER 4470/1/00 REV 1 CONVENT 47.
- Durkheim E (1953) *The Division of Labour in Society*. Free Press, Glencoe, IL.
- Elfant AB, Korn C, Mendez L, Pello MJ and Peikin SR (1995) Recall of informed consent after endoscopic procedures. *Dis Colon Rectum*. **38**: 1–3.
- Estey A, Musseau A and Keehn L (1991) Patient comprehension of printed health information. *Patient Educ Counsel*. **18**: 165–9.
- Faden R, Beauchamp TL and King NMP (1986) *A History and Theory of Informed Consent*. Oxford University Press, New York.
- Flesch RR (1948) A new readability yardstick. *J Appl Psychol*. **32**: 221–3.
- Flesch R (1949) *The Art of Readable Writing*. Harper and Brothers Publishers, New York.
- Fletcher CM (1973) *Communication in Medicine*. Rock Carling Monograph. Nuffield Provincial Hospitals Trust, London.
- Fletcher GP (1996) *Basic Concepts of Legal Thought*. Oxford University Press, New York.

- Fordham SD (1978) Increasing patient compliance in preparing for the barium enema examination. *Am J Radiol.* **133**: 913–15.
- Friedson E (1970) *The Profession of Medicine.* Dodd and Mead, New York.
- Gagliano ME (1988) A literature review of the efficacy of videos in patient education. *J Med Educ.* **63**: 785–92.
- General Medical Council (1998) *Seeking Patients' Consent: the ethical considerations.* General Medical Council, London.
- General Medical Council (2001) *Good Medical Practice May 2001.* General Medical Council, London.
- Gunning R (1952) *The Technique of Clear Writing.* McGraw Hill, New York.
- Gunning R (1968) The FOG index after twenty years. *J Bus Commun.* **6**: 3–13.
- Harpwood V (2001) *Negligence in Healthcare: clinical claims and risk.* Informa Publishing Group, London.
- Harris J (1985) *The Value of Life: an introduction to medical ethics.* Routledge, London.
- Hawkes N (2001) Nurse of the Year pioneers clinic. *The Times.* **31 October**: 3.
- Hawkins C (1985) *Mishap or Malpractice?* Blackwell Scientific Publications, Oxford.
- Henderson LJ (1935) Physician and patient as a social system. *NEJM.* **212**: 819–23.
- Holcomb CA (1983) The cloze procedure and readability of patient-oriented drug information. *J Drug Educ.* **13**: 347–57.
- Hynam KA, Hart AR, Gay SR, Inglis A, Wicks ACB and Mayberry JF (1995) Screening for colorectal cancer: reasons for refusal of faecal occult blood testing in a general practice in England. *J Epidemiol Commun Health.* **49**: 84–6.
- Jones WHS (trans.) (1967) *Hippocrates. Vol 11. Decorum XVI.* Heinemann, London (quoted in Polani PE (1983) The development of the concepts and practice of patient consent. In: *Convergence and Divergence in Tradition.* King Edward's Hospital Fund for London, London).
- Kanouse DE and Hayes-Roth B (1980) Cognitive considerations in the design of product warnings. In: LA Morris, M Mazzis and I Barofsky (eds) *Banbury Report 6: product labelling and health risks.* Cold Spring Harbor Laboratories, Cold Spring Harbor, New York.
- Katz J (1984) *The Silent World of Doctor and Patient.* The Free Press, New York.
- Katz J and Capron AM (1975) *Catastrophic Diseases: who decides what?* Russell Sage Foundation, New York.

- Kennedy I and Grubb A (1994) *Medical Law* (2e). Butterworths, London.
- Klare GR (1976) A second look at the validity of readability formulas. *J Read Behav.* **8**: 129–52.
- Lavelle-Jones C, Byrne DJ, Rice P and Cuschieri A (1993) Factors affecting quality of informed consent. *BMJ.* **306**: 885–90.
- Lear JT, Lawrence IG, Burden AC and Pohl JE (1994) A comparison of stress test referral rates and outcomes between Asians and Europeans. *J R Soc Med.* **87**: 661–2.
- Levy N, Landmann L, Stermer E, Erdreich M, Beny A and Meisels R (1989) Does a detailed explanation prior to gastroscopy reduce the patient's anxiety? *Endoscopy.* **21**: 263–5.
- Ley P (1992) *Communicating with Patients: improving communication, satisfaction and compliance.* Chapman and Hall, London.
- Ley P, Goldman M, Bradshaw PW, Kincey JA and Walker C (1972) The comprehensibility of some X-ray leaflets. *J Inst Health Educ.* **10**: 47–53.
- McCall Smith A (2001) Obtaining consent for examination and treatment. *BMJ.* **322**: 810–11.
- McKechnie S and Davies S (1999) Consumers and risk. In: P Bennett and K Calman (eds) *Risk Communication and Public Health.* Oxford University Press, Oxford.
- McKenna MC and Robinson RD (1980) *An Introduction to the Cloze Procedure. An annotated bibliography.* International Reading Association, Newark, DE.
- MacKinney LC (1952) Medical ethics and etiquette in the early Middle Ages: the persistence of Hippocratic ideals. *Bull Hist Med.* **26**: 1–31 (quoted in Polani PE (1983) The development of the concepts and practice of patient consent. In: *Convergence and Divergence in Tradition.* King Edward's Hospital Fund for London, London).
- McLaughlin H (1969) Smog grading: a new readability formula. *J Reading.* **22**: 639–46.
- McLean S (1999) *Old Law, New Medicine. Medical ethics and human rights.* Rivers Oram Press, London.
- Mason JK and McCall Smith RA (1999) *Law and Medical Ethics.* Butterworths, London.
- Mayberry JF and Fisher N (1989) Use of patient information booklet on inflammatory bowel disease by family practitioners. *Ital J Gastroenterol.* **21**: 53–4.
- Mayberry JF, Morris JS, Calcraft B and Rhodes J (1985) Information assessment by patients of a booklet on Crohn's disease. *Pub Health Lond.* **99**: 239–42.

- Mazzuca SA (1982) Does patient education in chronic disease have therapeutic value? *J Chron Dis.* **35**: 521–9.
- Meade CD, McKinney P and Barnas GP (1994) Educating patients with limited literary skills: the effectiveness of printed and videoed materials about colon cancer. *Am J Pub Health.* **84**: 119–21.
- Meredith P, Emberton M and Wood C (1995) New direction in information for patients. More attention should be given to finding out what works. *BMJ.* **311**: 4–5.
- Michielutte R, Bahnson J, Dignan MB and Schroeder EM (1992) The use of illustrations and narrative text style to improve readability of a health education brochure. *J Cancer Educ.* **7**: 251–60.
- Midgeley JM and Macrae AW (1971) Audiovisual media in general practice. *J R Coll Gen Pract.* **21**: 346–51.
- Mohammed M (1964) Patients' understanding of written health information. *Nurs Res.* **13**: 100–8.
- Moll JMH and Wright V (1972) Evaluation of the Arthritis and Rheumatism Council handbook on gout. *Ann Rheum Dis.* **31**: 405–11.
- Moll JMH, Wright V, Jeffrey MR, Goode JD and Humberstone PM (1977) The cartoon in doctor–patient communication. *Ann Rheum Dis.* **36**: 225–31.
- Mullen PD, Green LW and Persinger GS (1985) Clinical trials of patient education for chronic conditions. A comparative meta-analysis of intervention types. *Prev Med.* **14**: 753–81.
- National Health and Medical Research Council of Australia (1993) *General Guidelines for Medical Practitioners on Providing Information to Patients.* National Health and Medical Research Council of Australia, Canberra.
- NHS Litigation Authority (2000) *Clinical Risk Management Standards June 2000.* Clinical Negligence Scheme for Trusts, Bristol.
- NHS Management Executive (1990) *A Guide to Consent for Examination or Treatment.* NHS Management Executive, London.
- Nielsen E and Sheppard MA (1988) Television as a patient education tool: a review of its effectiveness. *Patient Educ Counsel.* **11**: 3–16.
- Parker CF (1981) Endoscopic movies for patient teaching. *AORN J.* **34**: 254–7.
- Parsons N and Glendening J (2000) The Human Rights Act 1998. Consent to treatment. *National Health Service Litigation Authority (NHSLA) Rev Issue.* **19**: 12–13.
- Pichert JW and Elam P (1985) Readability formulas may mislead you. *Patient Educ Counsel.* **7**: 181–91.
- Polani P (1983) The development of the concepts and practice of patient consent. In: GR Dunstan and MJ Seller (eds) *Consent in*

Medicine. Convergence and divergence in tradition. King Edward's Hospital Fund for London, London.

- Probert C, Frisby S and Mayberry JF (1991) The role of educational videos in gastroenterology. *J Clin Gastroenterol.* **13**: 620–21.
- Proctor DD, Price J, Mihas BS, Gumber SC and Christie EM (1999) Patient recall and appropriate timing for obtaining informed consent for endoscopic procedures. *Am J Gastroenterol.* **94**: 967–71.
- Rankin SH and Stallings KD (1990) *Patient Education: issues, principles and practices.* JB Lippincott, Philadelphia, PA.
- Redman BK (1992) *The Process of Patient Education.* Mosby Year Book, St Louis, MO.
- Rees JEP, Mayberry JF and Calcraft B (1983) What the patient wants to know about Crohn's disease. *J Clin Gastroenterol.* **5**: 221–2.
- Sanwal AK, Kumar S, Sahni P and Nundy S (1996) Informed consent in Indian patients. *J R Soc Med.* **89**: 196–8.
- Saw KC, Wood AM, Murphy K, Parry JR and Hartfall WG (1994) Informed consent: an evaluation of patients' understanding and opinion (with respect to the operation of transurethral resection of the prostate). *J R Soc Med.* **87**: 143–4.
- Schatzman L and Straass A (1955) Social class and moods of communication. *Am J Sociol.* **60**: 329–38.
- Schuck PH (1994) Rethinking informed consent. *Yale Law J.* **103**: 899–959.
- Smart H, Mayberry JF, Calcraft B, Morris JS and Rhodes J (1986) Effect of information booklet on patients' anxiety levels and consultation rates in Crohn's disease. *Pub Health Lond.* **100**: 184–6.
- Smith H (1946) Therapeutic privilege to withhold specific diagnosis from patient sick with serious or fatal disease. *Tennessee Law Rev.* **19**: 349.
- Snowman J and Cunningham DJ (1975) A comparison of pictorial and written adjunct aids. *J Educ Psychol.* **67**: 307–11.
- Stauch M, Wheat K and Tingle J (1998) *Sourcebook on Medical Law.* Cavendish Publishing Ltd, London.
- Switankowsky IS (1998) *A New Paradigm for Informed Consent.* University Press of America Inc., Lanham, MD.
- Taylor WS (1953) Cloze procedure: a new test for measuring readability. *Journalism Q.* **30**: 415–33.
- Trevelyan J, Needham EW, Halim M *et al.* (2001) Evaluation of patient characteristics and utilisation of invasive cardiac procedures in a UK ethnic population with unstable angina pectoris. *Int J Cardiol.* **77**: 275–80.
- United Kingdom Central Council for Nursing, Midwifery and Health Visiting (1996) *Guidelines for Professional Practice.* United

Kingdom Central Council for Nursing, Midwifery and Health Visiting, London.
- Wagenaar WA, Schreuder R and Wijlhuizen GJ (1987) Readability of instructional text written for the general public. *Appl Cogn Psychol.* **1**: 155–68.
- Weber M (1956) *The Protestant Ethic and the Spirit of Capitalism.* Scribner's, New York.
- Willows DM (1978) A picture is not always worth a thousand words. *J Educ Psychol.* **70**: 255–62.

Websites

British and Irish Legal Information Institute
http://www.bailii.org

BRI Inquiry: Final Report (July 2001)
The Inquiry into the management of care of children receiving complex
  heart surgery at the Bristol Royal Infirmary.
Bristol Royal Infirmary Inquiry Command Paper CM 5207.
http://www.bristol-inquiry.org.uk

Department of Health (2001)
Consent. What you have a right to expect. A guide for adults.
http://www.doh.gov.uk/consent/adultconsent.htm

Hungarian Civil Liberties Union
HCLU Policy Papers
Policy paper on the rights of patients.
http://www.c3.hu/~hclu/publ-3.htm

Koster N (1997)
Patient rights and patient education in The Netherlands.
http://www.nottingham.ac.uk/law/hrlc/hrnews/.../koster.ht

Patient Concern (2001)
How to survive surgery.
www.patientconcern.org.uk

Principles of the Rights of Patients in Europe (1994)
http://www.health.fgov.be/WH13/peri..../WWH19019804.ht

Cases

England and Wales

Blyth v Bloomsbury Health Authority [1987] ILR 9/2/1987: TLR 11/2/1987: [1993] 4 Med LR 151.

Bolam v Friern Hospital Management Committee [1957] 1 WLR 582–94.

Bolitho v City & Hackney Health Authority [1997] LTL 14/11/1997: TLR 27/11/97: [1997] 3 WLR 1151: [1997] 4 All ER 771: [1998] 1 Lloyd's Rep Med 26: [1998] 39 BMLR 1: [1998] 1 PNLR 1: [1993] 4 Med LR 381.

Breen v Baker [1956] *The Times* 27 January.

Re C (adult refusal of treatment) [1994] 1 WLR 290.

Caroline Smith v National Health Service Litigation Authority [2000] LTL 28/11/2000: [2001] Lloyd's Rep Med 90.

Chatterton v Gerson and another [1981] 1 QB 432–45.

Christine Williamson v East London and the City Health Authority and Others [1998] 1 Lloyd's Rep Med 6: [1998] 41 BMLR 85.

Elizabeth Ann Webb v (1) Barclays Bank plc (2) Portsmouth Hospital NHS Trust [2001] LTL 16/7/2001 (unreported elsewhere). Case No. B3/2000/2072/QBENF. Supplied by Smith Bernal Reporting Ltd for Lawtel 16/7/2001 (unreported elsewhere).

Re F (mental patient: sterilisation) [1990] 2 AC 1 HL.

Gillian Karen Carver v Hammersmith & Queen Charlotte's Special Health Authority [2000] QBD (Nelson J0 25/2/2000) LTL 10/4/2000 (unreported elsewhere).

Gillick v West Norfolk and Wisbech Area Health Authority [1986] AC 112.

Hamid Haghighat v Solicitors Indemnity Fund [1999] Supplied by Smith Bernal Reporting Ltd for Lawtel.

Heath v West Berkshire Health Authority [1992] 3 Med LR 57.

Hill v Chief Constable of Yorkshire [1989] AC 53.

Hills v Potter & Anor [1984] 1 WLR 641: [1983] 3 AER 716.

Re HIV Haemophiliac Litigation [1990] NLJR 1349.

Kunnath v The State [1993] 4 All ER 30: [1993] 1 WLR 1315: [1993] 98 CAR 455: Guardian 20/8/93: [1993] 137 SJ(LB) 195: [1993] 143 NLJ 1332: TLR 30/7/93.

Lloyds Bank plc v Waterhouse [1990] ILR 27/2/90: [1991] 10 Tr LR: [1992] 2 FLR 97: [1991] 2 Fam Law 23.

Re M (a minor) (medical treatment) sub nom. In the matter of the inherent jurisdiction sub nom re M (child: refusal of medical treatment) [1999] 2 FLR 1097: [1999] LTL 15/7/1999: [2000] 52 BMLR 124.

Norfolk and Norwich Healthcare (NHS) Trust v W [1996] 2 FLR 613.

Re MB (Caesarean section) [1997] LTL 26/3/97: ILR 8/4/97: TLR 18/4/97: [1997] 2 FLR 426: [1997] FCR 541: [1998] 38 BMLR 175.

Pearce v United Bristol Healthcare NHS Trust [1999] 48 BMLR 118.

Re R (a minor) (wardship: consent to treatment) [1991] 4 All ER 177, CA (Lord Donaldson MR, Staughton and Farquharson LJJ).

S v S [1970] 3 All ER 107.

Sidaway v Bethlehem Royal Hospital Governors [1985] AC 871, HL at 871: [1984] 1 All ER 1018, CA: [1985] 1 BMLR 132: [1984] QB 493.

Slater v Baker and Stapleton [1767] 8 Geo 111 860–63.

Smith v Tunbridge Wells Health Authority [1994] 5 Med LR 334 339 QBD (Morland J) (25/5/95).

Re T (adult medical treatment without consent) [1992] 4 All ER 649 CA 30/7/92.

Re W (a minor) (medical treatment) [1992] 4 All ER 627, 633.

Scotland

Moyes v Lothian Health Board [1990] 1 Med LR 463, [1990] SLT 444.

Other jurisdictions

Arndt v Smith [1997] 2 SCR 539.

Canterbury v Spence [1972] 464 F. 2d 772, 784 (D.C. Cir. 1972).

Cooper v Roberts [1971] 220 Pa. Super. 260, 286 A.2d 647.

Hondroulis v Schumacher [1989] 553 So 2d 398 (La. 1989).

Hopp v Lepp [1980] 2 SCR 192 at 210.

Malette v Shulman [1990] 72 OR 92d 417.

Mohr v Williams [1905] 104 NW 12.

Natanson v Kline [1960] 350 P.2d 1093 (Kan. 1960).

Pratt v Davis [1906] 118 Ill. App. 161 224 Ill 300, 79 NE 562.

Reibl v Hughes [1980] 2 SCR 880, 114 DLR 93d 1 14 CCLT 1, Can SC.

Rogers v Whitaker [1992] 175 CLR 479, 109 ALR 625, 16 BMLR 148.

Rosenberg v Percival [2001] 178 ALR 577.

Salgo v Leland Stanford Junior University Board of Trustees [1957] 317 P.2d 170, 181 (Cal. Dist. Ct. App. 1957).

Schloendorff v The Society of the New York Hospitals [1914] 211 NY 125, 105 NE 92.

Truman v Thomas [1980] 165 Cal. Rptr. 308, 611 P.2d 902 (Cal. 1980).

Walsh v Irish Family Planning Services [1992] 1 IR 496.

Statutes

Health Care Consent Act 1996, S.O. 1996

Medical Liability and Insurance Improvement Act of Texas, 1979, Art. 4590i. Vernon's Texas Civil Statutes

Mental Health Act (1983)

National Health Service and Community Care Act, 1990

Public Health (Control of Diseases) Act 1984

The Human Rights Act 1998

The Patient's Right to Know Act of 1996, Florida

The Uniform Consent Law of 1990 (R.S. 40: 1299.40E), Louisiana

Information sheet about gastroscopy

Gastroscopy

Why do I need this test?

A gastroscopy allows your doctor to examine your gullet (or oesophagus), your stomach and your duodenum. It is used to find out the cause of stomach pains, weight loss and bleeding. It can pick up inflammation, ulcers and tumours.

How is the test done?

The test is done with an *endoscope*. This tube is a camera. It can make a video of the inside of your gullet, stomach and duodenum. The stages in the test are as follows.

- Your mouth is sprayed with local anaesthetic. This will make it numb.
- You can choose to have the test done under sedation. This will make you relaxed but *not* asleep. The test is *not* usually done under a general anaesthetic.
- The endoscope is passed over the back of your tongue and into your gullet.
- Your stomach and duodenum are then examined with the endoscope.
- It is likely that several small samples of tissue will be taken during the test. These are called *biopsies*.

How long will the test take?

The test is unlikely to take more than 10 minutes. The results from some biopsies can be ready in 20 minutes. Most biopsies need to be prepared in a laboratory. This will take several days.

How safe is the test?

The test is very safe, but there are risks. The main risk is that the endoscope can tear the gullet or stomach. This can happen about once in every 3000 tests. If this happens it may need to be repaired with an operation.

Questions

Please tick the right answers.

		True	False
1	The endoscope can be used to find the cause of indigestion.	☐	☐
2	The test is usually done under a general anaesthetic.	☐	☐
3	The test usually takes less than 10 minutes.	☐	☐
4	The test is perfectly safe and never has any risks.	☐	☐

Further examples of information sheets

Further examples of information sheets with an associated test, based on the gastroscopy model, are given. One is for a flexible sigmoidoscopy and the other is for a colonoscopy.

The basic principle illustrated by these three 'test' sheets is that they should check that patients understand:

1 the purpose of the test or procedure
2 the risks associated with the procedure
3 the type of sedation used with the procedure and its mode of action
4 its likely duration.

Incorrect answers allow the clinician to identify areas where the patient has failed to understand the test or procedure. He or she can then discuss this aspect in greater detail.

The sheet should carry a patient identification label and be filed as part of the clinical record. The sheet should be signed by both patient and clinician and record further discussions where misunderstandings have been clarified. As such it can form a permanent part of the clinical record.

An example of a patient choice information sheet

In a number of clinical situations there are alternative methods of investigation or of undertaking the procedure. In the case of gastro-scopies, patients may choose no sedation, intravenous sedation or a general anaesthetic. Indeed there are other possibilities such as acupuncture or hypnosis. A barium meal may be a less effective test, but again is an alternative method of investigating the upper gastrointestinal tract. Doctors and nurses are expected to discuss alternatives with patients. At present such choices are seldom documented in detail in the clinical record. However, an example of a possible anaesthetic decision tree for patients in endoscopy is presented as a way of ensuring that patient decisions are properly documented and annotated.

Flexible sigmoidoscopy

Why do I need this test?

A flexible sigmoidoscopy allows the doctor to examine the lower part of your bowel. It is used to look for the cause of diarrhoea or constipation. It can also find the cause of rectal bleeding and anaemia. It can pick up inflammation, polyps and tumours.

How is the test done?

The test is done with a *flexible sigmoidoscope*. This tube is a camera. It can make a video of the bowel. The stages in the test are as follows.

- You can choose to have sedation. This will make you relaxed but *not* unconscious. The test is *not* usually done with a general anaesthetic.
- Your bottom will be examined internally with a finger by the doctor. This relaxes the bottom. It also allows the doctor to feel an area which the camera examines poorly.
- Your lower bowel is then examined with the flexible sigmoidoscope.
- It is likely that several small samples of tissue will be taken during the test. These are called *biopsies*.
- Polyps are small tumours. They are usually benign. They can be removed during the test. This is done with an electrical cutting method.

How long will the test take?

The test is unlikely to take more than 10 minutes. Any biopsies or polyps will be examined in a laboratory. This will take several days.

How safe is the test?

The test is very safe, but there are risks. The main risk is that the sigmoidoscope can tear the bowel. This can happen about once in every 3000 tests. If this happens it will need an operation to repair the hole. The risk is greater if you need to have a polyp removed.

Questions

Please tick the right answers.

		True	False
1	The sigmoidoscope can be used to find the cause of anaemia?	☐	☐
2	The test is usually done under a general anaesthetic?	☐	☐
3	The test usually takes less than 10 minutes?	☐	☐
4	The test is perfectly safe and never has any risks?	☐	☐

Topics of further discussion

. . . .

. . . .

. . . .

Signed: . . . . (patient)

            . . . . (endoscopist)

Date: . . . .

Colonoscopy

Why do I need this test?

A colonoscopy allows the doctor to examine the lower part of your bowel. It is used to look for the cause of diarrhoea or constipation. It can also find the cause of rectal bleeding and anaemia. It can pick up inflammation, polyps and tumours.

How is the test done?

The test is done with a *colonoscope*. This tube is a camera. It can make a video of the bowel. The stages in the test are as follows.

- You can choose to have sedation. This will make you relaxed but *not* unconscious. The test is *not* usually done with a general anaesthetic.
- Your bottom will be examined internally with a finger by the doctor. This relaxes the bottom. It also allows the doctor to feel an area which the camera examines poorly.
- Your lower bowel is then examined with the flexible colonoscope.
- It is likely that several small samples of tissue will be taken during the test. These are called *biopsies*.
- Polyps are small tumours. They are usually benign. They can be removed during the test. This is done with an electrical cutting method.

How long will the test take?

The test is unlikely to take more than 20 minutes. Any biopsies or polyps will be examined in a laboratory. This will take several days.

How safe is the test?

The test is safe, but there are risks. The main risk is that the colonoscope can tear the bowel. This can happen about once in every 3000 tests. If this happens it will need an operation to repair the hole. The risk is greater if you need to have a polyp removed.

Questions

Please tick the right answers.

1 The colonoscope can be used to find the ca
   anaemia?
2 The test is usually done under a general a
3 The test usually takes less than 20 minutes?
4 The test is perfectly safe and never has any risks?

Topics of further discussion

. . . .

. . . .

. . . .

Signed: . . . . (patient)

        . . . . (endoscopist)

Date: . . . .

...ion and gastroscopy

...gastroscopy can find the cause of your symptoms. The test takes 5 to 10 minutes. It can be done with sedation or without it. This leaflet describes the types of sedation which can be used. You can choose which sedation you would like.

The test can be done with:

- **No sedation** – you will be fully awake for the test.
- **With sedation** – you will feel relaxed. You will *not* be asleep.
- **A general anaesthetic** – you will be totally unconscious. You will need an extra visit to hospital to check on your fitness for this anaesthetic.

Before the test you can also have a **mouth and throat spray** which will numb feelings in your mouth during the test.

Mouth and throat spray

Some people find holding a toothbrush in the mouth makes them feel sick. If this happens to you, you may find the gastroscope has a similar effect. You may then choose to have a mouth and throat spray. This makes the mouth numb.

What is the spray?

The spray is a local anaesthetic. It is called lidocaine. It is said to have a banana flavour, but many people say it tastes 'horrid'.

How is the spray given?

The spray may be given to you by a nurse or a doctor. Between 1 and 20 sprays are made into your mouth. You will be asked to swill the spray around your mouth for up to 30 seconds. You will then be asked to swallow the spray.

The effect of the spray lasts from 12 to 45 minutes. **You must not eat or drink during this time.**

What are the risks of the spray?

Complications are uncommon. However, the spray can cause:

- feelings of anxiety
- breathing problems
- loss of consciousness.

Must I have the spray?

No. There are several studies which have shown that many people have the test done easily without the spray.

SEDATION

Firstly, a small tube is placed in a vein in the hand or elbow. Sedation is given by injection into this vein. Two sedatives could be used. They are:

- diazepam
- midazolam.

These drugs are similar. They both can:

- relieve anxiety
- cause you to forget unpleasant memories of the test.

Their side-effects can include:

- deep sedation
- sexual fantasies
- interference with normal breathing.

Diazepam is mild but long acting and can cause drowsiness for several hours.

Midazolam is shorter acting but more likely to cause deep sedation and so breathing problems. Very rarely this can cause death.

GENERAL ANAESTHETIC

If you want a general anaesthetic for your test, you will have this done on a different date. You will need to be admitted as a day case and seen by a nurse and an anaesthetist. They will confirm that you are fit for an anaesthetic.

A general anaesthetic will ensure that you are completely asleep for the test. All general anaesthesia carry a risk. However, the risk of death is very small at less than 1 in 100 000 anaesthetics given.

YOUR CHOICE

For your gastroscopy which do you want?

Mouth and throat spray

I would like:

No spray ☐   Lidocaine spray ☐

Sedation

I would like:

No sedation ☐   Sedation by vein ☐   General anaesthesia ☐

If you would like sedation by vein would you like it to be:

Diazepam ☐   Midazolam ☐   Either, I will leave ☐
the choice to the
doctor

Reactions to medicines

Sometimes people know they have had a reaction to certain medicines in the past. This could have been at the dentists or in hospital. Have you ever had a reaction to:

	Yes
Lidocaine	☐
Diazepam	☐
Midazolam	☐

Signed: . . . .

Date: . . . .

Index

Index entries are to page numbers, those in italic referring to Tables. Where legal cases are referred to but only named in the end-of-chapter notes, the reference is to the page number followed by 'n' and the number of the relevant end-of-chapter note.